SOME REVIEWS

The Cancer Path

Everyone wonders how they would confront cancer, should they develop it. Let Paulette Sherman be your guide. This is an inspiring account of her experience of breast cancer demonstrating courage, wisdom, resilience, and insight, told with love, compassion, and understanding.

LARRY DOSSEY, MD
AUTHOR OF *HEALING WORDS, REINVENTING MEDICINE*, AND *THE ONE MIND*

Paulette Sherman writes her beautiful story of healing, resilience and love. Read this book and discover how to conquer even your worst fears with love.

EVA SELHUB, MD, AUTHOR OF *THE LOVE RESPONSE*

When we can love our fate and learn from our journey through hell, in one form or another, we become life coaches for others. Paulette's experience can help guide you through the journey into cancer land and help you to find the path which will guide you out and learn how to be a survivor.

BERNIE SIEGEL, MD, AUTHOR OF *FAITH, HOPE & HEALING* AND *HELP ME TO HEAL*

One does not know cancer until you experience it. The initial fear of the unknown shocks you into isolation and helpless. I understand this as the husband of a breast cancer survivor. And I also know that the courage from our spiritual nature brings hope and the resolve to fight. Paulette Sherman has described this beautifully in her struggle and victory. Her story of fear, spiritual healing, love and mind/body interventions is an outstanding plan for those in need.

DR. JAMES D BAIRD, AUTHOR OF *HAPPINESS GENES*

The Cancer Path is more than one woman's journey through cancer; it is the most thorough guide I've ever read about navigating the cancer experience. This is the book I wish I'd had to guide me when I went through the cancer experience myself.

Randy Peyser, author of *The Little Book of Big Epiphanies* and *Bald Courage*

As a physician, I have great admiration for people such as Paulette Sherman, who continue to live their best life despite their personal health obstacles and work hard to support others facing similar circumstances. I am so inspired by Paulette's courage and positive energy, her resilience and ability to take all her challenges in stride. Her step by step, holistic approach is sure to be immensely helpful to those struggling to cope with a diagnosis of cancer.

Karen Levine-Tanco, MD, Beth Israel Hospital

Dr. Paulette Sherman demonstrates the power of spirituality and inner wisdom in dealing with difficult challenges in life. Illness is a spiritual journey and Paulette's experience is an inspiring witness to the power of spirituality in each person's life—in health and in illness. The book should be read by health professional students, for it reminds all caregivers to honor the whole person—mind, body and spirit.

Christina M. Puchalski, MD, Physician
author of *Time for Listening* and *Caring and Making Healthcare Whole*,
Professor of Medicine, Director, The George Washington University's
Institute for Spirituality and Health (GWish)

Paulette was able to describe with a lot of sentiment her experience in the dramatic situation of breast cancer. She was able to transform the sadness of this experience into a positive feeling that she can transmit to other women in the same condition.

Dr. Virgilio Sacchini, Breast Surgeon at Sloan Kettering Hospital

There has never been a more thoroughly written book on breast cancer. Paulette has detailed not only the real life experience of living with and surviving the cancer but also outlines in detail all the options available to women as they search for the best options.

Dr. John Salerno, The Salerno Center, author of *The Silver Cloud Diet*

With the understanding befitting a psychologist and the chatty tone of your best friend, Sherman empowers her readers! Comprehensive, creative, practical and rich with resources, *Cancer Path* offers something for everyone!

Susan Silberstein, PhD, author of *Hungry for Health* and *Hungrier for Health*, Founder, Center for Advancement in Cancer Education

Paulette Sherman's moving story about her new life after cancer inspires all cancer survivors and, what is more, gives all of us powerful ideas and tools—like yoga—for handling any challenge in life.

Tari Prinster, a cancer survivor and yoga teacher
author of *Yoga Prescription: Using Yoga to Reclaim Your Life During and After Cancer*, Founder of yoga4cancer and The Retreat Project

For most of my life I have taught about the 'dark night of the soul' and how each and every person goes through this transformational process at least once per lifetime in one form or another. Paulette Kouffman Sherman has been through this process in the form of cancer and survived to tell about it. There are only two ways we can all go through our 'dark night' . . . the easy way or the hard way; *The Cancer Path: A Spiritual Journey into Healing, Wholeness & Love* offers the reader some clear and insightful methods for turning even the most difficult path into a journey of love, healing, and personal mastery.

—Michael Mirdad, Bestselling Author, *Healing the Heart & Soul* and *You're Not Going Crazy . . . You're Just Waking Up!*

The Cancer Path

A Spiritual Journey into Healing, Wholeness & Love

by Dr. Paulette Kouffman Sherman

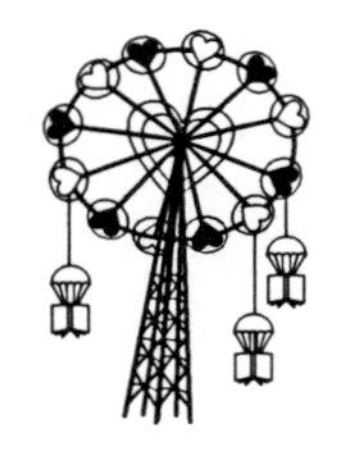

Parachute Jump Publishing®
"Books that inspire you to l♡ve more"

Parachute Jump Publishing
www.ParachuteJumpPublishing.com

Parachute Jump Publishing paperback edition, April 2013
Manufactured in the United States of America
Designed by Sara Blum
Edited by Margie Holt Smith & Wendy Thornton

Sherman, Paulette Kouffman.
The Cancer Path: A Spiritual Journey into Healing, Wholeness & Love / Paulette Kouffman Sherman; foreword by Ana Negron.

LCCN 2013900189
ISBN - (paperback) 978-0-9852469-4-5
1. Illness 2. Spirituality.
3. Memoir. I. Title.

This is my love letter to the world

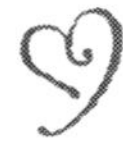

I have sent you nothing but angels—God

Neale Donald Walsch

This book is dedicated to my sister Avra & her boyfriend Albert, who travelled a long way to visit me on two occasions and stayed for two weeks during my treatment-and showered me with unconditional love and healing

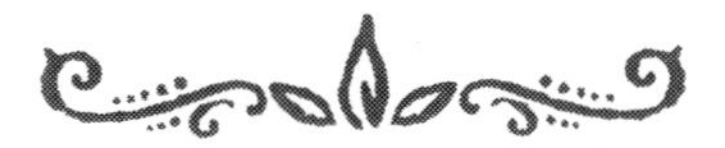

Table of Contents

SECTION II

SECTION III

SECTION IV

Foreword

Without a doubt the diagnosis of breast cancer creates a traumatic shift in any woman's life. Her wisdom, flooded with anxiety and fear, may fall out of reach at a time when she needs it most. This is why I am so relieved that my friend, Paulette Kouffman Sherman, allows us to follow her. She leads her readers from one milepost to the next, gathering many tools along the way. She creates links to wise ones among us through their quotes. She assures us that playfulness is serious business.

Written during one of a woman's most difficult journeys, we walk at Paulette's swift pace through her cancer treatment and have no choice but to share in her openness and hope. In many passages you will hear the unmistakable voice of a mentor, a guide, a wise companion, prompting us to engage in life more fully.

This book is more than a memoir. It is a reminder of our resilience. While every year over two hundred thousand women in this country are given the diagnosis of breast cancer, millions continue to survive it. Paulette and this book help us braid together many strands of healing.

Without a doubt the diagnosis of breast cancer creates a traumatic shift in a woman's life. Her wisdom flooded with anxiety and fear may fall out of reach at a time when she needs it most. This is why I am so relieved that Paulette would let us follow her. She leads her readers from one mile post to the next gathering for us many tools. She creates links to wise ones among us through their quotes. She assures us that playfulness is serious business.

Paulette and I both know that when a person must accommodate to sustained toxic levels of stress, such as occurs when navigating the churning waters of our not always logical or caring health care system, she uses up vital defenses. Short bouts of stress turn stasis into motion, but many people regard increasing levels of stress and worry as normal.

Lucky for us, one of Paulette's many skills is cutting to the chase without wasting precious energy. Wallowing in indecision is not her style. We have much to learn from her approach to obstacles and to the unknown.

Throughout her career, Paulette has helped people practice more authentic lives and develop more meaningful and loving relationships. Her lifetime of work becomes even more important when a woman is called to be in a meaningful and loving relationship with herself. The healing work is not over at the last chemotherapy treatment.

When we negotiate on our own behalf, no holds are barred. Yet women may be the hardest sell for this notion. These days, love and compassion seem in short supply. In my thirty-five years practicing family medicine, I have seen how hard women judge themselves. Super caring women often fall into states of vulnerable exhaustion and still don't even recognize this has occurred. As a woman places herself in the hands of her trusted medical team for whatever treatment she decides, she must also quiet the inner voices and listen to herself. Healing cannot take place without her. This is her story. I believe that the work Paulette has put before us is as inspiring as the life of each of us.

One of the gems in this book is the promise of transformation. Whether we go willingly or thrashing and cursing, both are legitimate ways into more life. Redressing the way we live may be the very last medicine left for us to drink. We can turn the stark path ahead into a rich, illuminated trail where wholeness and love reign.

Ana M. Negrón, MD
Wayne, Pennsylvania
www.greensonabudget.org

Introduction

Everything that happens to you is a gift. There is a kernel of beauty in everything if you have the eyes to see it.

FORTUNE FROM A THAI RESTAURANT

It was the day before my 41st birthday and my doctor had some news: I had triple negative (stage 2) breast cancer.

And there was a twenty-five percent chance of recurrence.

I barely had time for my regular life. With two kids under 4, full time work, a 90 minute commute and trying to write a book . . . cancer just wasn't a good fit for me. No thanks.

But the rabbit hole opened and I was sucked in, seemingly against my will. Down I fell, like a parachuter landing in the Amazon with no map and no experience of the territory. I scrambled to get my bearings and to reroute my plan. Using all my senses, slowly, I felt my way around and soon they began to open up.

In the darkness, a divine light inside of me began to shine and I looked within instead of trying to conquer the outer world. My journey reminded me of the story that I once heard about the Rainmaker. He was sent to a town experiencing a drought. His job was to make it rain, but when he got there he put up a tent and sat inside for a long while. When he came out, he made it rain. Someone asked him why he went into the tent first and he replied that the outer conditions were imbalanced so he had to go within to become aligned before he could affect the outside world. To me, my tent was symbolized by the triangle of Mind/Body/Spirit. I needed to create an inner balance before I could ever hope to affect outer change, in my own condition and perhaps in the health care system as well.

My cancer journey was like Alice in Wonderland, where every experience and person led me somewhere new. I had to be open to learning and growing. It was like a dream sequence where all the characters were like a part of me—some were too serious, cynical, or scientific—where I became friends with the angels and learned how to banish my demons and even face death so that I could love life, myself, and others more.

My 1 ½ year-old-daughter Sera epitomizes joy and laughter even at the most stressful of times. She has no concept of time or what's appropriate: she is just pure joy. Some nights we'll finally be asleep at 3 a.m. and she'll wake up and do a jamboree singing performance in her crib in the dark and start laughing. One time my tired husband yelled at her and she cried. It broke my heart to see the light in her eyes temporarily dim. But then, fifteen minutes later she had forgotten and was singing her heart out again—loud, clear, and unafraid.

I guess it's our job as adults to get back to that type of unmitigated insane inner joy, despite our outer circumstances and obstacles, because that's who we really are.

We can learn how to let go and let God in. This cancer journey helped the Divine in me play, speak, and roar, culminating in this book and in my own healing journey. I used to have everything reasoned and measured. Now it can be felt with my heart.

I've detailed healing tools that can help you on your way. This book documents how cancer triggered an inner journey in me, which revealed itself as a spiritual path. This spiritual path then expressed itself in my relationships, work, self-care, healing, and values. And now that I've recently graduated from the school of cancer, I consider myself a pathfinder and guide who can help you navigate your own path. I have tracked my own trail and I am now encouraging you to discover your path of revelation. There's a labyrinth here with a center of completion, yet you may find yourself wandering in and out in discovery. This confusion, advance, and retreat is part of the process of learning and healing. And hopefully this book will remind you that you are not alone. I'd love for you to be healthier and happier than you were before cancer so you feel that travelling this path is worth it. It was to me!

And although the banana split sundaes I used to enjoy have been put on hold since my cancer diagnosis, I've found a new sweetness that's lasting and long. It's in the delighted song of the angels who take things lightly and make everything holy. May you too find the magic to heal and live within these pages.

And remember: in this state of grace and inspiration, all is divine. Work is play and surrender can become a co-creation with life itself. Cancer is a spiritual path and initiation, if you choose to see it that way. I hope you will join me in surrendering as we dance together down this Cancer path: a spiritual journey into healing, wholeness and love.

My Best in Love and Light,

Paulette

Develop a Powerful Context for Your Cancer

He who has a why to live for can bear almost anyhow.

NIETZCHE

When I first got cancer, I was dumbfounded. Why me? I thought.

I was just trying to accept it, deal with it, and keep everything going.

I was lucky to have my sister and her boyfriend from California come stay with me for two weeks when I was first diagnosed. My sister was my grounding rod. She said she didn't want to leave me without support and structure, what with two kids and working full time while living in the middle of Coney Island! She suggested angel healers, and before she left, she *insisted* that I call this guy she knew from California, Chris. She wanted me to promise that I'd be positive and would create a support structure instead of just working hard and being stoic.

I called Christopher Dilts, who I like to call "my angel guy." He gave me a spiritual context for what was happening. I wanted to make meaning of my experience, to learn from it and to turn it into something inspiring. I was hopeful that it happened for a reason, and Chris agreed.

When I first found out about the cancer (before talking to Chris), I asked my Higher self how I'd feel if I were to die. I was told that I had accomplished most of my dreams. I had work I loved and helped many people, I'd married the love of my life, had two beautiful children—a boy and a girl, lived on the beach, and had published a few books. But then my Higher Self said, "You still have to publish 22 books. This is also your legacy."

Twenty-two books?" I thought! *"But I'm exhausted!"* The thought of trying to get an agent and a publisher felt like a lot of work. So right then I decided to self-publish instead and to just "put my books in the river." If my messages of love were "out there" then the right people could find them, I'd have fulfilled my mission and I'd be fully expressed. Writing was no longer an ego issue; it was just something I loved. I decided to let go of the results.

Chris confirmed this Legacy project, saying that I should tell myself that "my mission is stronger than my cancer."

I tell you this because viewing my cancer as a spiritual experience that held important lessons was a turning point for me. It elevated the experience from a random occurrence of suffering and punishment to an opportunity for my soul to grow and contribute.

You can attempt this if it feels true for you, enlisting the help of a spiritual mentor like Chris or by just spending some time with your Higher self and asking questions about why this is happening and why you are here. Everyone's answers will be individual.

I have written this book to help others view cancer as a spiritual path, but within that context, everyone's journey will be unique.

Healing Cancer From the Inside Out

True healing and miracles must take place in the heart and soul before actually reaching the body.

Michael Mirdad

The reason I've included the body, mind, emotions, and Spirit aspects of healing in this book is that there is a feedback loop between them. If you change your thoughts (mind) this can affect your emotions and your nervous system (body). If you perform deep breathing exercises and this affects your body, it can also affect your mind and emotional state. With cancer and any illness, there are two phases to the journey: what heals you and what helps you to cope throughout treatment and the final solution to an illness and the longer journey to wellness and maintaining it. When we treat symptoms and not the underlying causes then the illness can pop up again. We need to address any imbalances in our mental, physical, emotional and spiritual energies to explore any root causes of which we may be unaware. I would highly recommend addressing your stress, self-care and balance during your treatment. A good way to do this is to put together a healing team to address your mind/body/soul and Spirit.

As you will see throughout this book, I strongly suggest that you approach healing yourself on all these four levels, so you can address the source of the disease and not just the symptoms. The next four sections of this book will address the mind, body, emotions and Spiritual aspects of your healing and energy body. At best, I hope to inspire you to further explore on your own. Maybe I can save you from reading 60 books (as I did) while you are undergoing your treatment *and* trying to take good care of yourself. Hopefully you will get a lot of condensed preliminary information here by just reading this one book!

There will be starts and stops with most treatments; at least, there were for me. So prepare yourself for disappointment with some healers that cross your path. Some will not get back to you or they will drop out without explanation midstream. Also, alternative treatments can get expensive because usually health insurance won't pay for alternative healers, which is a challenge.

In later sections we will look at alternative therapies and healers, what worked and what didn't (at least for me as the guinea pig). Also in these sections, I will examine contrary information from both sides of different issues. This is tough to do when you only have two weeks as a patient to first absorb your diagnosis, decide and arrange your medical treatment path, and to try to figure out the best holistic treatment plan. I hope to make things easier by providing this overview for you, and remember, your treatment will probably last 8 months to a year, so you do have time.

My first book in this Cancer Path series, *The Quick Guide to Breast Cancer: Diagnosis, Surgery, Chemo & Radiation*, explores tips and preparations to help cancer patients complete their standard cancer treatment in a straightforward manner. If a patient wants to go deeper and heal themselves on all four levels, questions emerge that are confusing. Healers say different things so a patient has to weigh all sides and decide for herself. When you're already confused or overwhelmed, you are hoping that the path is at least somewhat clear and the research and experts all point in one direction. But . . . no such luck with cancer!

Whether it's about diet, stress, the cause(s) of illness or even getting a henna crown or drinking green tea and taking antioxidants, you will get fierce and intelligent opposition from each side. And as exhausted as you are, you probably won't have energy to research the information much before making a decision yourself. So, I have tried to do some of this work for you, describing both sides of some important issues as best I could (as a patient), allowing you to then choose your own path in the 3-4 week window that you are usually given before beginning your treatment. And as I mentioned, I've read well over 60 books so that hopefully you can just read this one!

Here's an example of dissenting opinions. The one thing I thought I knew was that in cancer, *your immune system* breaks down! I figured that when I was done with my treatment, I'd need to do things to build my immune system back up. Tons of alternative healers believe this too. But when I spoke to my radiology oncologist, he said they don't think that cancer is caused by a poor immune system because AIDs patients do not have a greater incidence of breast cancer and their immune system is down. When I asked him further about this, he said they really don't know what causes cancer because only a small percentage is genetic. I later read somewhere that many people with normal immune systems develop cancer and many people with damaged immune systems don't.

In *The Journey Through Cancer*, Dr. Jeffrey Geffen explains that since cancer cells arise from within our body, it's hard for the immune system to tell the difference between a normal cell and a cancer cell. And if the immune system can't distinguish which cells to kill, then simply boosting your immune system may not help. So, here's an example where as a patient you think, *"So, is the immune system important at all, or not?"*

There may not be a clear, definitive answer yet (or irrefutable proof). So if it's not contra-indicated to build your immune system *after* your chemotherapy and radiation treatment, why not do so? Patients want to do things that empower them to heal themselves.

To further complicate matters, some doctors will tell you to wait until *after* your treatment to build up your immune system because it will interfere with their chemotherapy and radiation goals, whereas others will say to build your immune system throughout the process. I chose the former approach because I was afraid of messing up the effects of the chemotherapy and radiation and I certainly didn't want to go through *that* again! Doctors will tell you to eat regularly, skip juicing, and not take supplements during chemotherapy.

In the chapters that follow, we will explore other confusing treatment issues like: Does diet matter? Does stress affect your immune system? Does your emotional state and your overall vibration affect your cells? Can resentment contribute to getting cancer? Do energy and chakras affect your health? Can cancer be a spiritual calling? Can alternative therapies help heal cancer and how? How can your loved ones support or hinder your progress? Does the balance of mind, body, emotions and Spirit make a difference in your long-term healing? Can having the right healing team support your recovery? How can you best advocate for your own care? The following sections, divided into Body, Mind, Emotion and Spirit are the only linear parameters on this winding cancer path.

I don't want you to think you can pray or meditate and cure your cancer. I am not a medical doctor, and as I've already said, there is no clear proven explanation or understanding of cancer at this time. So as a patient (like you) I aim to maintain a balance between medical and spiritual perspectives, to empower you to weigh all the information for yourself, and to improve your overall health and life. Having recently been down this road I can tell you what worked best for me on my path toward healing, wholeness, and love.

I explore my personal experience along this Cancer path with snapshots to help you reflect personally, and with exercises to work through if you so choose. I introduce information from the many books I read during this time as milestones. I suggest that as you read this book, you circle the sections with information or exercises that you may want to return to, although you never know what surprises will arrive and take you off in another direction.

As you go through each section of the book, notice whether you feel most out of balance in the body, mind, emotions or Spirit categories and begin there. Remember, balance brings with it wholeness, healing and peace.

I hope that by joining me on this cancer path you will find answers within yourself so you can join in the discussion about what creates greater love, peace, and healing in your own life during and after cancer.

So, let's begin!

SECTION I

Body

Just when the caterpillar thought the world was over, it became a butterfly.

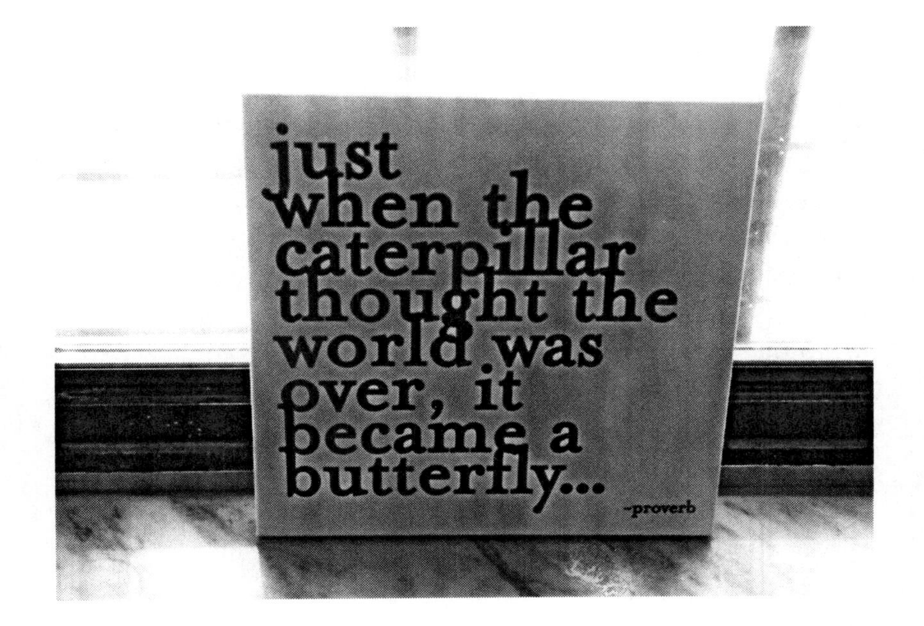

A SIGN IN MY ROOM

Your Body Image

This is a call to arms. A call to be gentle, to be forgiving, to be generous with yourself. . . When the criticism drops away, what you will see then is just you, without judgment, and that is the first step toward transforming your experience of the world.

Oprah Winfrey

If you were already someone who didn't feel great about your appearance, then having breast cancer can really throw you for a loop. The most obvious change in appearance from cancer is losing all your hair, often including your eyelashes and eyebrows. For some women the idea of being bald may seem like the ultimate insult to your sense of desirability and attractiveness. But of course, as we know, when you are dealing with a potentially life-threatening illness you do rearrange your priorities, and temporarily baldness may hurt our vanity but it is survivable! Plus, you get to play with wearing wigs—a great chance to change your "do" and take on other, fun personas.

Personally, I wasn't too concerned with how I looked when baldness happened to me. I used to pay greater attention to my looks when I was single and dating, but since becoming a married, working, mother of two children, I barely had time to look in the mirror anyway. Plus, my sense of self-worth didn't hinge on externals so much any more.

So, I was able to deal with my baldness with a sense of humor and to take my lumpectomy scar in stride. I think it was also easier to not get so upset about outside cosmetic changes because I have a husband who loves me no matter how I look—or at least says he does, and I believe him!. I am grateful for that.

It may sound a little weird but after a while I just ditched the wigs and felt kind of cool bald. I felt like a monk or priestess. In a strange way the baldness made me feel lighter and more confident. I liked to wear dangly earrings, which added a dash of femininity, and I often wore an electric blue liquid eyeliner that really brought out the Egyptian goddess in me and hid the fact that I had no eyelashes. When my eyebrows fell out, sometimes I'd fill them in with a brow pencil, sometimes not. Sometimes I wore silver sparkly sneakers with my hospital gown because they made me (and other patients) smile. So, remember, you are beautiful from the inside out, and you can always come up with creative ways (scarves and hats can be fun, too) to feel more confident and feminine during this process. What you tell yourself about your self-image has a lot to do with how great you can feel.

When I was receiving treatments at Sloan Kettering hospital I took a free class called "Look Good, Feel Better," that I would recommend to you. It's a two hour class that teaches you to do your eyebrows and apply makeup that is appropriate for your skin tone. There are similar classes at most hospitals and you can call 1-800-395-LOOK to find out where this class is offered if it isn't at your hospital. It's fun, good for your vanity, and you're given free makeup and professional instructions on makeup application.

Perhaps an unexpected gift in all these physical changes is that you can learn how to feel beautiful in a new way, from the inside out. You may notice how your eyes sparkle or that you love your smile, instead of focusing on your hair or eyelashes. You may realize that beauty radiates from within. Ironic that in losing all my hair I became more aware of my inner and outer beauty, and took more time to look in the mirror and appreciate who was looking back at me.

When I had my mammogram at the lab, they put a pretty pink sticker on my lumpectomy scar. These stickers are pink, pretty and fun, and they peel right off. They match the scar perfectly. To order these **special scar stickers** call: *Beekley Medical* S-Spot for Mammography Skin Stickers. They are a thin row of pink flowers, like a removable scar tattoo!

While at Beth Israel's West Side Mind/Body/Spirit library one day, I discovered a wonderful book about your "image" during cancer treatment called *Facing the Mirror With Cancer*, by Lori Ovitz with Joanne Kabak. I've put it in the reference section and you can order it if you need extra help with maintaining your looks during treatment. Remember that you are loveable no matter what you look like.

So, I was mostly okay with my image. I decided to let go of my hair in stages, and had cut it short prior to losing it all. Random people would compliment me on my haircut, as though I'd chopped it off because I desired a short haircut. Funny. But I won't kid you, there were days I looked awful and I knew it. One week, on a day that I was supposed to meet my husband's new boss and co-workers at a special "meet and greet" I woke up that morning with three cold sores! I was also supposed to be interviewed in a video, which fortunately I could postpone to the following week. I asked my husband to snap this picture with my phone so that I could show you, so hopefully you won't feel alone when you have your not-so-great days:

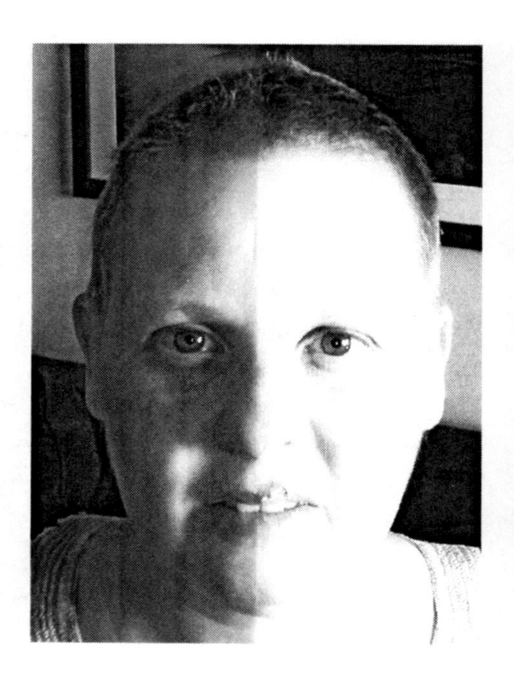

After waking up and peering in the mirror, I wandered into the living room and said, "I look terrible for tonight's event!" My 4-year-old son, Noble, was sitting on the couch watching his cartoons and he replied, "You don't look terrible. You look like a princess!" I could have kissed him (but didn't want to give him my cold sore). Hopefully you will have someone like this in your life too. If not, you can always pretend that you do.

Ladies, his sweetness totally cheered me up. My adorable, wise, son makes a good role model for all the husbands, boyfriends, and friends of women on the cancer path to up their compliments to you on those days when they're most needed. And, you can always compliment yourself!

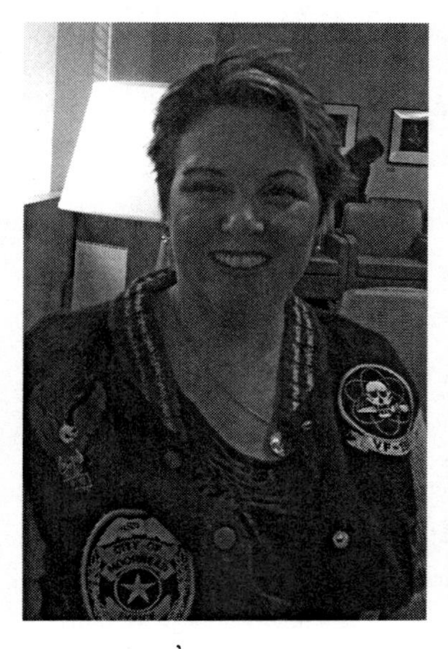

HERE'S ME WITH A SHORT HAIRCUT

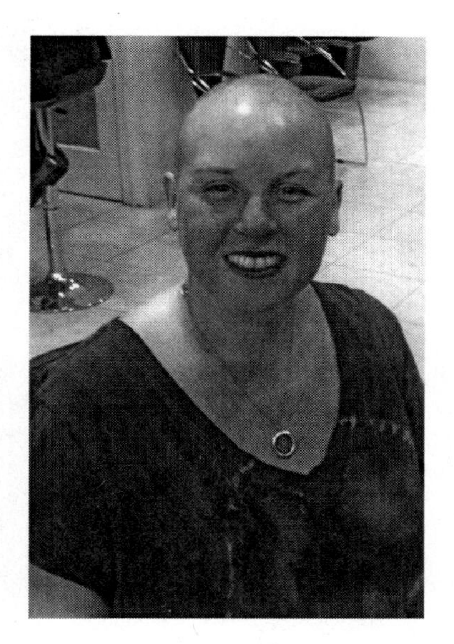

ME BALD

Then one day (after chemo #2) it started to fall out in clumps. I decided just to go to my hairdresser and shave it off. This is me bald, something I thought I'd never see.

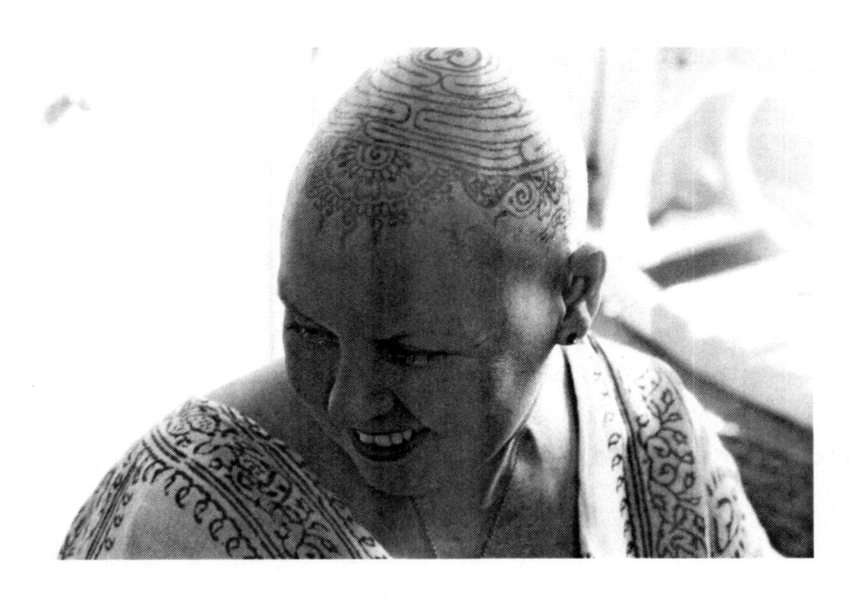

HENNA CROWN

Next I visited a few wig places in my area. I loved red hair, so my wig was my chance to be a red head.

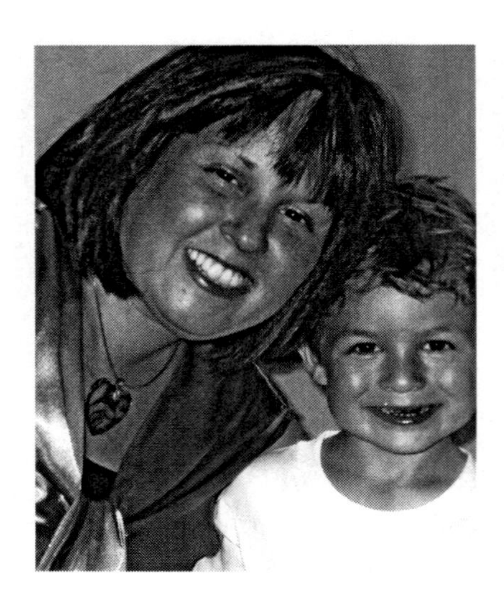

ME IN MY NEW LONGER SYNTHETIC WIG, WHICH WAS TOO HOT!

Another thing I did to cheer myself up was to get a henna crown. When I was at Sloan Kettering hospital my oncologist told me not to get a henna crown because she said there was not enough research in support of it while I was doing chemotherapy. But when I switched hospitals to Beth Israel, my oncologist Dr. Malamud said he was okay with it because henna was ancient and it had been around for years. I was so happy just to hear yes about something a bit out of the box that I thought might help me!

Henna crowns are a great option for women who lose their hair from chemo. I heard about it through an organization called www.hennaheals.org. They referred me to a henna artist in NYC named Kenzi. She came to my house and created my henna crown. I will put Kenzi's number in the Resource section of this book if you're in New York, but you can also Google henna artists near you.

Many of these artists do Indian or Moroccan henna designs. I wanted to create a labyrinth with a heart in the middle of my head with some butterflies and flowers, representing growth, transformation, and my spiritual cancer path. So, you can create your own design or use traditional symbols. Henna art will last one to two weeks.

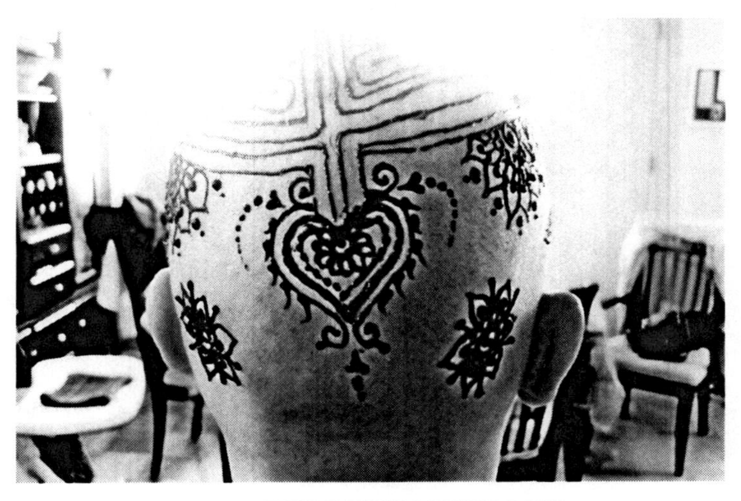

HENNA WHILE IT WAS BEING DONE

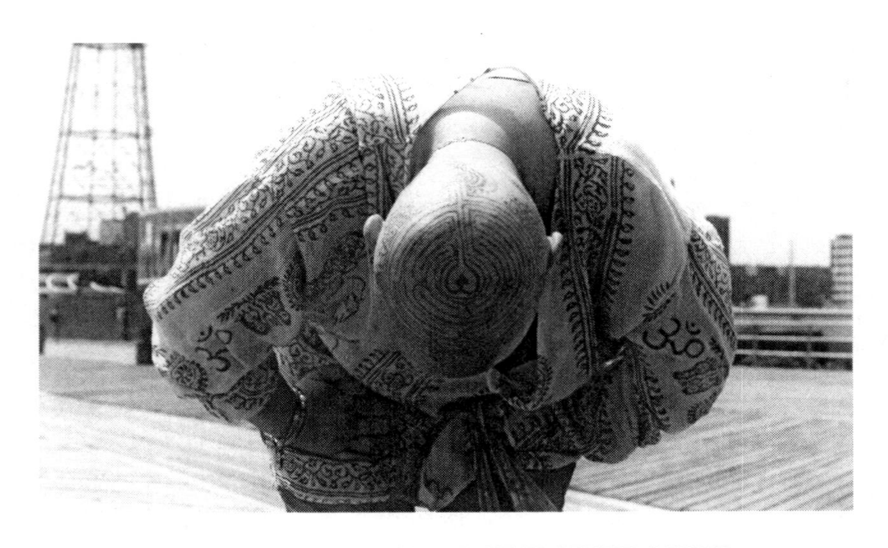

MY CANCER PATH WITH HEART IN CENTER DESIGN

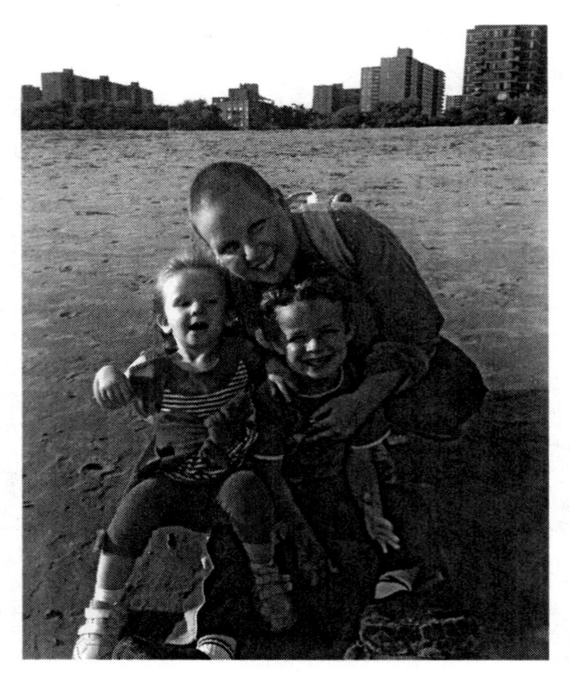

MY PEACH FUZZ HAIR WITH MY KIDS ON THE BEACH

Your Relationship with Your Body

As a body everyone is single, as a soul never.

Hermann Hesse

As I said, I was estranged from my body and didn't take much time to pay attention or listen to it. Even as I write this advice, I realize that I still don't take much time to nurture my body or hear the wisdom from that part of myself. So, I'm writing this subsection for my benefit as well.

If your body has become out of balance with illness, stress or disease, it may have a message for you. You can take some time to close your eyes, breathe deeply and meditate, asking it what it needs. It may be good to have a journal on hand to record the wisdom you receive. It may say, *Slow down. Sleep more. Feed me more live foods like fruits and vegetables. Play or move more.* It may not be anything fancy. Perhaps something simple is missing and can make a big difference in your overall health should you be willing to really listen and reintegrate that energy. This might mean changing your habits and priorities. Maybe this is why many of us tune it out. But cancer is one way our body gets our attention and says, "Wake up!"

A simple and powerful exercise is to write a letter to your body, allowing the response to flow through you as automatic writing. For example:

Dear Body,

Why did you get breast cancer? Are you trying to tell me something? I'm listening . . .

Sheila

(response)

Dear Sheila,

I am tired from all your running around and you helping everyone but yourself. I know you think you are doing good but you are running me into the ground and I need healing, love, and rest. You need to reprioritize and put me–our–wellbeing first! I'd also like to have more fun please! Stop ignoring me! You need me and I love you.

With Fierce Love,
Your Body

Try this for yourself. You may be surprised by what you hear. This is a chance to reconnect and start a lifelong dialogue. Let your body tell you how you're doing. Don't just wait for the doctor until something is wrong.

ENERGY TESTING

Another way to become more attuned to your body is *Energy Testing*. In her book, *Energy Anatomy*, Donna Eden describes how energy testing (also known as muscle testing) allows you to determine whether an energy pathway is flowing or blocked, and whether an organ is getting the energy it needs to function, and whether an outside energy is harmful to your system. This tool allows you to ask your body what it needs. You can ask questions about medications, treatment, foods, vitamins, supplements and environmental choices best suited for your body. Eden believes that the medical profession would be helped by adding energy testing as a diagnostic tool for determining the choice and dosage of medications. Research has shown scientific support for this method and Eden says energy tests consistently support what she sees in a person's energy fields.

I have not yet used this tool but I would like to take a class on muscle testing. It seems easy to learn and many of you may find it sufficient to learn and practice energy testing simply by reading the instructions in Eden's book. This can be one more tool to keep in your toolbox to help you attune to what your body wants and needs, and to make health-positive choices along your cancer path.

PREVENTATIVE AND AFTERCARE

Eden also talks about *preventative care for your breasts*. Since you, dear reader, most likely already have/had breast cancer, you can try this exercise after your treatment ends. I won't go into detail but the exercise is self-massage to stimulate lymph fluids to flow freely and drain lymph fluid from the breasts. (You can find this exercise on page 279 of *Energy Medicine*.) She suggests that you use this massage technique each time you remove your bra to keep the energy flowing in your breasts and to keep them healthy. Underwire bras, so popular in modern societies, do us a disservice, clogging the neurolymphatic points there and inhibiting energy flow: resulting in slow, steady harm to the lymphatic tissue in the breast. Clogged energy there can create pain and an internal environment that invites future health problems, including cancer.

In *The Complete Cancer Cleanse*, Cherie Calbom writes that wearing a bra fourteen hours a day increases the hormone prolactin, which causes decreased circulation in breast tissue. She cites research by medical anthropologist Sidney Singer who compared the incidence of breast cancer in two groups of women in the Fiji islands. One group of women wore bras and the other did not. Those who wore bras had the same breast cancer rate as American women but those who did not wear bras experienced almost no breast cancer. Calbom recommends that women remove their bras as much as possible and don't sleep with them. Donna Eden prefers nursing bras and suggests wireless bra brands like Sassybax, Abundantly Yours, Vanity Fair style 532, Expectant Moment #4426, Victoria Secret's no wire IPEX wireless bra, and Just My Size.

Eden also says that working with the Houston valve and ileocecal valve can help with nausea and digestive problems. So if you have those symptoms after chemotherapy, check out pg. 281 in her book for suggestions about this issue.

The next section on body will explore your nervous system, diet, chakras, movement and other healing techniques for your body.

Your Central Nervous System

Your function on earth is healing.

A Course in Miracles

According to Donna Eden, "Your nervous system is a phenomenally sensitive thirty-seven mile long antenna that reverberates to the subtle and not-so-subtle energies of the world in which we live." There are two parts of your central nervous system: the *sympathetic* and the *parasympathetic* nervous system.

The *sympathetic* branch of your autonomic nervous system originates in the spinal cord. It goes into action to prepare the body for physical or mental activity. In response to a stressor, the sympathetic nervous system orchestrates what you familiarly call the fight-or-flight response. It increases muscle blood flow and tension, dilates pupils, accelerates heart rate and respiration, and increases perspiration and arterial blood pressure. Chronic stimulation of the *sympathetic nervous system* disturbs systems, increasing health risks like gastrointestinal problems, immune system problems, cardiovascular and endocrine issues.

The *parasympathetic nervous system* conserves energy and maintains the body's homeostasis, producing relaxation. You can activate the parasympathetic nervous system through meditation, visualization, deep breathing and progressive muscle relaxation.

There is a converse relationship between these two systems. When the parasympathetic nervous system goes up, the sympathetic goes down and vice versa. This is often an unconscious process but we want to try and be aware whether we are creating or exacerbating fight or flight conditions (aka stress), or if we are creating relaxed states in our body—via our thoughts, etcetera. Every time you notice that are in "fight or flight" mode you can do something to help you relax and return to your parasympathetic nervous system.

This book will provide specific tools and techniques that tend to stimulate your parasympathetic nervous system, which is also the best mode to access your Higher self, divine wisdom, and healing on the levels of mind, body, emotions and Spirit.

Sleep

Sleep is God. Go worship.

JIM BUTCHER

Sleep was difficult the first three days, due to the steroids I took during chemotherapy. My body was so tired but my energy level was too high to sleep. I was given Ativan to take at my discretion for nausea and to help me sleep, but I felt like I was already taking so much medication that I chose not to take it. You can ask your doctor what to do to help you sleep ahead of time, and you may choose to take additional medication. Sometimes I would toss and turn and get hot flashes due to the chemotherapy. I usually found by the third or fourth day after chemotherapy I was so tired that I could finally sleep.

I also listened to angel healing tapes that my sister had brought me from California. They were tapes by LaUna Huffington. I will put the ordering information in the Resource section. My husband would make fun of me, but I found her voice very soothing, healing, and sleep—inducing, so you may want to try that for yourself, or listening to dolphin or ocean music.

Remember, your sleep is a very important aspect of your health plan. According to Dr. Amy Lowry of Sloan Kettering Hospital, 10%

of the general population has sleep problems lasting three months or more, and with cancer survivors the rate is three times higher!

Also, sleep may be helpful for preventing recurrence. Researchers at University Hospital's Case Medical Center in Cleveland, Ohio, showed an association between insufficient sleep and biologically more aggressive tumors. Thompson's study showed the hazard of too little sleep for women who already have cancer. Participants with six hours of sleep or less per night had higher tumor recurrence scores. In an article by Angelina Tala called, "Lack of Sleep, Light at Night Can Raise Cancer Risk," the author found that 70% of Americans are not getting the average hours of sleep they need. However, women who sleep 9 hours a night have a 70% lower breast cancer risk!

Research shows that blind women have 50% less breast cancer than sighted women. They live in darkness 24 hours a day and sleep more than the average American sighted woman, producing higher levels of melatonin and cortisol. Melatonin is an antioxidant thought to fight cancer cells and it needs darkness.

Dr. Richard Stevens, a cancer epidemiologist and professor at University of Connecticut Health Center, has researched how electric lighting at night may cause circadian rhythm disruption and hormonal changes. Stevens said the more there is darkness, the more melatonin gets produced and the lower the cancer risk. He performed a study on lab rats where two groups of rats were injected with breast cancer causing agents. One of two groups was injected with melatonin and studies showed that the melatonin in rats prevented them from getting breast cancer. Stevens doesn't advise taking melatonin tablets, though. He says staying in the dark at night is better. He also feels that electric lights, cell phones, computers, etc. change our hormonal rhythms and may contribute to breast cancer rates.

Sleep is also when your body repairs itself at the cellular level, and the body's circadian rhythm is interrupted during poor sleep. Researchers say we do much better with at least eight hours of sleep, and cancer clients going through chemotherapy ultimately need more sleep and naps so their body can repair and rest. Keeping the same sleep and wakeup time every day is optimal for our health and circadian rhythm.

My husband and I have two walking alarm clocks that automatically wake us up at 6 a.m.—our two kids! This means that I had to do my best to go to sleep by 10 p.m. to get eight hours sleep. Sometimes both kids wake up at night but there's nothing to do about this. I found some things that helped me to sleep, including taking a bath, putting on my angel meditations and music, making the room dark, and mentally leaving my "to do" list until morning.

Take a moment to note how much sleep you are getting and what might improve your sleep. As I said, during chemo I was given Ativan to take as needed, but I never took it. If you want to explore pharmaceutical possibilities, ask your doctor. You can also ask your doctor if you can take a natural supplement like tryptophan to make you drowsy.

There was one night where my mother-in-law babysat our kids at her house, and my husband and I slept the night through from 9 p.m. – 9 a.m. It felt like a miracle to get 12 hours of sleep! I could feel how much my body needed it. Maybe a family member can help you out this way.

Especially when you take steroids during chemo you may find it hard to sleep through the night. It doesn't help that you may be getting hot flashes, nausea, or headaches. I found it helpful to read in bed or sometimes to eat something like a banana to address the nausea.

My neighbor and health coach, Dan, had insomnia for many years until he got some orange-blue blocking sunglasses. He says that 45% of our brain is sensitive to light signals. According to Dan, the blue-green light stops our brain's production of melatonin, the hormone that helps you sleep. Neurosurgeon Jack Kruse agrees that melatonin is one of the most powerful brain antioxidants, and it clears our brains of inflammatory junk. Dan says that the orange glasses balance the blue light and since he has worn them, he sleeps for 10 hours! You can purchase these glasses for $50-$80 normally, but Dan found a pair for

$8 on Amazon. Be sure they are 99% orange. I did not need to try this but it might be something helpful for you to try. I've included more information on these glasses in the Resource section.

We need rest to refuel. Author Donna Eden says, "Your body forces you to slow down so it can rebalance, release toxins, and regenerate itself in the energy-restorative magic of sleep."

Getting adequate sleep is one very enjoyable change to make, so you may want to begin your self-care there with sleep aids.

Movement, Body Work and Other Good Things for Your Body

Movement never lies. It is a barometer telling the state of the soul's weather to all who can read it.

Martha Graham

Research shows that exercise significantly reduces the risk for cancer, the risk of recurrence, and the risk of death associated with cancer. The greatest risk reduction was found in women who exercised 10 - 19 hours per week, or two hours a day for five days, but even light intensity exercise like walking reduced their risk. A study done on triple negative cancer showed that exercising four times a week reduced recurrence. Cancer survivor and author Kris Carr says that the body heals 8 times faster with exercise because exercise floods your body with oxygen and gets rid of toxins via your lymphatic system.

Breast cancer survivors are among the least physically active cancer survivors. They are only about half as active as women who have not had cancer. According to Prijatel in *Surviving Triple Negative Cancer*, research published in the *Journal of the National Cancer Institute* showed that low levels of exercise and high body mass index were risk factors for triple-negative cancer. Of most significance was weight gain between the ages of 35-50 and a body mass index of above 31. Exercise was a more potent deterrent for hormone-negative cancer than hormone-positive cancer because women who exercise are more likely to have lower levels of insulin in their blood and are more likely to maintain a normal body weight. Prijatel mentions a scary statistic in her book, citing that the Collaborative Women's Longevity Study found that women who gained more than 22 pounds after diagnosis were 83% more likely to die of breast cancer than those who stayed within 5 pounds of their original weight. Also, women increased their death risk 14% for every 11 pounds they gained after diagnosis!

The *Journal of Sports Sciences* (March 2009) reports that moderate or vigorous exercise reduced breast cancer risk by 44%. In 2007, the journal *Cancer Detection and Prevention* showed that breast cancer risk was reduced by 40% among women with moderate physical activity and 57% with vigorous activity. A study published in the April 2009 issue of the *International Journal of Cancer* linked increased physical activity with decreased risk of death with breast cancer. Moderate-intensity exercise decreased the risk of breast cancer recurrence, progression, or development of a new primary cancer.

Researchers at Colorado State University have suggested that physical activity decreases breast cancer risk by muscular, hormonal, and metabolic mechanisms. The findings from a large, well-respected study of U.S. nurses, found that breast cancer patients who walk or do other kinds of moderate exercise for three to five hours a week are about 50 percent less likely to die from the disease than sedentary women. I also read that trampoline jumping is great for stimulating your lymphatic system. So is a jump rope or any exercise that requires you to bounce up and down. Walking on the beach was my favorite form of exercise. I decided that I am going to start slowly though, and I'm noticing that I am drawn to very feminine forms of movement instead of things that require brute force and discipline. I was more tired through the chemo so I needed things that were easy, like walking in nature or yoga.

Author Sonia Choquette says that movement and exercise affects you spiritually, raising the vibration of the body and flushing negative energies, and making a clear space for the soul to return. Choquette also writes, "You cannot aspire to higher levels of consciousness until you are peaceful in your present physical awareness. Your body is the best teacher because it precisely reflects how you are viewing yourself." Her statement piqued my interest, to think of the body as another path to spiritual development instead of just a flesh container. How does your body pre-cancer or post-cancer reflect how you are viewing yourself?

What follows are different types of movement and body work that are gentle and can be appropriate to include in your well-being plan as you go through your treatment, and beyond.

YOGA

For thousands of years yoga was practiced as a physical discipline toward a spiritual path. Popular today for its effectiveness in reducing anxiety and enhancing energy, millions of people have found that yoga in subtle and profound ways significantly improves one's quality of life. A recent study at the M. D. Anderson Cancer Center examined just this: the use of a yoga program in improving the quality of life in women undergoing radiotherapy for breast cancer. Results indicated statistically and clinically significant quality of life improvements for these women.

In March 2010 a review of studies on yoga for patients with cancer was published, which included 10 trials. The studies determined that yoga could help to reduce anxiety, depression, fatigue and stress for some patients. And it improved the quality of sleep, mood and spiritual well-being for some people.

I took a yoga class with yoga teacher and cancer survivor Tari Prinster, who became a yoga teacher after her diagnosis of breast cancer. She had done yoga before her diagnosis but reports it was mainly for cosmetic reasons then. After diagnosis it became a powerful inner tool and journey. She used yoga practice as a powerful tool to manage the daily challenges of cancer treatments and the side effects. Eventually she became a yoga teacher and focused her practice on proactively managing the lifelong vulnerabilities cancer treatments can create. She developed a unique, carefully constructed system of yoga poses and sequences based on the specific needs of cancer survivors. In 2003, she began teaching a yoga class for cancer survivors and offering workshops and retreats. With that grew the need and interest in a yoga teacher certification utilizing her researched methodology. She has since trained over 450 yoga teachers from all over the world to meet the physiological and psychological needs of this special population. Her "Yoga 4 Cancer" classes are designed to address the needs of cancer survivors and patients, provide safe healing yoga, and provide a community where cancer survivors can bond with others "touched by cancer." Tari lectures on yoga and cancer and launched *The Retreat Project*, a non-profit that funds annual retreats for low-income and under-served populations, endeavoring to encourage and cultivate access to the transformative power of yoga. She has an upcoming book called, *Yoga Prescription: Using Yoga to Reclaim Your Life During and After Cancer.*

DANCING

Dancing to your favorite songs or singers can be very invigorating, even if you only dance for 10 minutes. It gets your adrenaline pumping and makes you feel great. You even get the added benefit from singing along, as most of us like to do. If you want to make dancing a communal activity you can dance with your kids or spouse. We used to have a disco ball with a spotlight in our living room, which was a lot of fun. Plus, dancing is easy to do and you need no props and can do it anytime in your house! No need to feel silly or that you "can't dance," just let go and express yourself. There is a parallel process here between physical, emotional and spiritual wellness.

WALKING

Walking synchronizes the brain, gets your heart rate up, builds bone density and is great exercise. It's free and you don't need any props for it, plus you can appreciate nature and the outdoors.

I live by the beach, so my favorite form of exercise during treatment, and afterwards, was (and always has been) walking. The added benefit of movement and walking in nature inspires my soul. Walking is an ideal form of exercise for many people since it requires no props and can largely be done anywhere or any time. I found that since I could temper the pace according to how I felt on any given day, it was ideal exercise throughout my treatment. If walking is appropriate for you, I encourage you to get out in nature as much as possible: the beach, a park, a pond, or river. You can take a friend with you but it's also great to go alone so that you can connect with yourself and hear any inner or nature-inspired divine guidance. Sometimes I'd also take my iPhone and headphones and plenty of angelic meditations or beautiful music to accompany me. This is a great way to set the tone and your consciousness for your day.

If you would rather walk indoors, a good dvd is *Walk Slim* by Leslie Sansone. She has positive energy and it's easy to do it at home.

REIKI

Reiki is a light touch, hands-on treatment that encourages the body to achieve mental, emotional, physical, and spiritual balance. It can reduce anxiety and pain too.

Human energy flows through meridians in the body. A disturbance in the flow of this energy may be caused by physical illnesses or negative emotions. Reiki practitioners channel universal life energy to problem areas in the client's energy flow where it is sensed as being disrupted. The Reiki practitioner aims to move and balance the energy within and around your body, and to remove any "energy blocks" to physical healing and strengthening of the individual's energy. The Japanese word for the universal energy, *Ki*, is used to describe the universal life energy being worked with in Reiki. Reiki practitioners believe that therapeutic effects are obtained from *Ki*, which they learn how to channel through them, and provides strength, harmony, and balance to the body and mind.

Practitioners believe that Reiki can treat symptoms and improve mental clarity, well-being, and increase your spirituality by making you feel more connected to universal energy. It has been proposed that Reiki can lower heart rate and blood pressure, boost the immune system and endocrine (hormonal) systems, stimulate endorphins, or affect skin temperature and blood hemoglobin levels. However, these properties have not been well-studied or clearly demonstrated in scientific studies yet.

A Canadian phase 2 study in 2003 examined whether Reiki could control pain in people with advanced cancer. Subjects did report a significant reduction in pain after Reiki treatment, but the results are based only on a study of 20 patients. Many cancer patients I know have reported that Reiki relaxes them and decreases pain.

I decided that if Reiki wasn't painful I might as well try it. I found it to be very relaxing, and lucky me, I had a high school friend who was getting her Reiki certification and needed practice hours, so she gave me two Reiki treatments at my house! Thanks Rachel.

I learned that other hospitals *do* integrate Reiki with good results, even for surgery. Reiki practitioner Raven Keyes was the first Reiki master to practice in an operating room, under the supervision of Dr. Mehmet Oz. She worked with Dr. Oz at Columbian Presbyterian

Hospital and with Dr. Sheldon Feldman, a doctor who works with breast cancer patients. Dr. Feldman reports that when Raven does Reiki during surgery, the patients' blood pressure remains steady, they need less pain medication after surgery, and the patient does better overall in recovery. Raven wrote a book about her experience doing Reiki for healing called, *The Healing Power of Reiki* (which I will put in the Bibliography section for you).

In spite of my unremarkable experience with self-administered Reiki at Beth Israel (the full story is detailed in Book 1: *My Quick Guide Through Breast Cancer*), practitioners do advise you to take a Reiki certification course and get "attuned" so you can give yourself a treatment daily for free. This seems like too much to take on during cancer treatment, but maybe afterwards. There are also Reiki circles offered in many communities that are inexpensive. In Manhattan, The Open Center offers a Reiki certification for all 3 levels. You can look for a similar holistic center near you. You can also check around and see if any friends offer Reiki, and your hospital may offer it as well.

My friend Rachel recommended that I speak to her Reiki teacher Joanna Crespo.

Joanna had DCIS herself (which was stage 0 breast cancer, almost stage 1). Doctors suggested that she have a mastectomy but she did not need radiation or chemotherapy. She had a plastic surgeon do the reconstruction of both breasts, which took a year to finish.

She coped like a good soldier, but when she saw her breasts without nipple tattoos she broke down and cried: the loss felt deeply and unexpectedly personal. Everyone had just assumed that she was fine by that point and they had moved on. Her husband pretended that cancer didn't exist, her mom nagged her, and others put up a brave front on her behalf. So, Joanna coped with a lot of her feelings alone. Her right breast became hard (encapsulated), so she had to have additional reconstruction surgery to correct this. Soon her doctors will tattoo her nipples, and hopefully that will be the last surgery for her.

Joanna took 4 weeks off to stay home after her surgery and then 2 more weeks off for her first reconstruction. Many people offered to do Reiki on her but this felt intrusive to her at the time because she felt they saw her as "cancer" and wanted to "do something to her." An older Reiki practitioner that Joanna knew called her and was very matter-of-fact, saying that she wanted to come to her house the day before her surgery to perform Reiki healing. Joanna agreed, so this woman did so, and she also went to the hospital to give Joanna and the other patient in her room Reiki, the day after surgery. Joanna remembers that their room had a great energy and she was up and about after her surgery. For her, Reiki helped with the pain and healing.

Joanna says that she would not have gotten through this experience without her own self-Reiki practice though because it helped her so much to hear her Spirit. Joanna realized that on a physical level she developed cancer because her cells had to adapt when they lacked oxygen. Joanna reported this because she had read that cancer cells develop when they lack sufficient oxygen. This realization allowed her to make her peace with Cancer, and this took away her fear of it. But since she had practiced Reiki before finding her breast cancer diagnosis, she realized that Reiki can't protect you from Cancer because Cancer is life. And Joanna feels that Reiki is a spiritual practice that helps you cope with life.

I asked Joanna how Reiki might help breast cancer patients. Joanna says that for her, Reiki supplied spiritual energy to connect with divinity, so she could open herself up to be filled with love. She says that sometimes when she does this practice she can feel a divine presence that fills up every atom in the room. Ultimately, Joanna says, the healing is between the client and their ability to listen to the divine, and it is that relationship which does its own healing work. She has learned that the more you practice Reiki, the more intuitive you become, and a client's body will often tell you where your hand should be placed. Joanna feels that Reiki can lead people to their own truth, since it is another discipline that opens you to a Higher power.

I asked her whether Reiki helped her to find an emotional cause to her breast cancer and whether she believed in that concept. She said that she thinks breast cancer is often about mother issues, either with your parental mother, or related to nurturing yourself. She describes herself as someone who was often caught up in her own head rather than connected to her heart. When her own Reiki teacher died of colon cancer she was angry at her, but this experience moved her from her being predominantly in head and into her heart, and ironically, this prepared her to deal with her own breast cancer later, coming full circle.

Today, Joanna knows that love is the creative force that drives everything. Reiki can help people engage divinity in aligning their intention and thoughts with love so that they can find a better path to healing and wholeness.

ACUPUNCTURE

Acupuncture can be helpful for cancer patients, particularly with symptoms of anxiety and nausea. Studies show it can help with peripheral neuropathy and hot flashes. The World Health Organization lists more than 50 medical conditions for which acupuncture is effective.

Acupuncture works with the meridian system. The meridian network is described as 24 pathways that carry energy into, through, and out of your body. Points along these pathways can be stimulated with needles or you can use physical pressure (acupressure) to release and redistribute the energy. Each segment is named for the organ it serves. The meridian network transmits information from one part of the body to another and it is the underlying template for the physical body. Eden describes the meridians as the body's energy bloodstream, which can determine the speed and form of cellular change. It is important to be aware of this energetic aspect of ourselves but often we are not taught about it.

In a *NY Times* article by Tara Parker-Pope called, "Acupuncture Offers Relief for Breast Cancer Patients," research revealed that acupuncture was helpful for symptoms of hot flashes, sweating, and lack of energy. Research from the Henry Ford Hospital in Detroit, presented at the American Society for Therapeutic Radiology and Oncology's meeting in Boston, studied acupuncture use among 47 women who were receiving anti-estrogen treatments, including Tamoxifen or Anastrozole (Arimidex). These drugs are known to lower the risk of breast cancer recurrence, but they can also trigger menopause-like symptoms, including hot flashes and night sweats. Half the women were given the antidepressant Effexor. The other half received acupuncture therapy once or twice a week during the 12-week study.

Findings showed that the acupuncture worked just as well as the antidepressant Effexor to curb hot flashes. Women who received acupuncture reported fewer side effects and more energy, and some reported an increased sex drive, compared to women who used Effexor.

I tried acupuncture three times when I was going to the "You Can Thrive Foundation." I was a bit weary of needles but it didn't really hurt and I felt good afterwards. I had a woman in my yoga class who said that having weekly acupuncture sessions helped considerably with her symptoms, so it may well be worth looking into for you as well. It would be great if more health insurance companies would cover acupuncture treatments for patients. This may be the case in the future, and currently some health insurance companies do offer it, so check. There are also acupuncture schools where staff-supervised students will treat you at low or no cost. Make sure that you tell them that you are undergoing chemotherapy and that the school is a professional institution.

TAPPING, OR EFT

A popular trend is called *tapping*. Tapping helps shift self-defeating patterns of thought and behavior. Tapping was developed based on applying acupuncture principles to psychological issues. Acupuncture is associated with needles but you can also tap, hold, or massage acupuncture points, or even apply heat to them. At least 360 acupoints are distributed along the network of meridians. David Feinstein and Donna Eden say that if you can shift energies you can influence your health, emotions, and state of mind. I would recommend their book, *The Promise of Energy Psychology*, which details how to use energy techniques like tapping to shift anxiety, depression, and other psychological issues.

Feinstein says that our brain consists of one hundred billion neurons that connect electromagnetically with up to ten thousand other neurons in governing your energy, movement, feeling, and thought. Tapping works physiologically by holding a triggering image/painful experience in mind, while physically stimulating a series of acupoints that send impulses directly to the amygdala, which inhibits the alarm response. These impulses cause a reduction within the amygdala of the number of neural connections between the image and the alarm response, which doesn't change the memory but the emotions connected to it.

Feinstein explains that psychological and behavioral habits are embedded in your energy system, neurology, and lifestyle. Energy psychology focuses on the energy disturbance as well as the memory. The basic ETF recipe, according to David Feinstein, involves rating the amount of distress when you bring a specific thought or memory to mind. Then you tap on acu points to decrease the emotional charge around that thought or memory by making a statement acknowledging the problem, and at the same time affirm that you accept yourself with that problem. While you make this statement you work with some of the points to move energy through your body.

Some examples of statements would be:

Even though I am overweight,
I deeply love and accept myself.

Even though I am not eating healthy,
I deeply love and accept myself.

Even though I am worried the cancer will return,
I deeply love and accept myself.

Even though I am still overworking,
I deeply love and accept myself.

You can find the basic tapping sequence of 8 points in the book, *The Promise of Energy Psychology* (pg. 43).

There are many books and tapes you can get to teach yourself this tapping technique, which is also sometimes called EFT or Emotional Freedom Technique. Although I did not learn it during my cancer path I still would like to take a class to use it as an additional healing tool. I figure it can't hurt for you to try it and many people have found it to be very helpful. For some more background on tapping, purchase the DVD, *The Tapping Solution*. You can also find free tapping demonstrations on YouTube.

MASSAGE

Studies show that massage can improve circulation, enhance sleep, reduce stress, tension and pain. It's also a way to give yourself love during a challenging time.

My dad did a very sweet thing. He paid for three 30-minute massage vouchers and then renewed them. Near my office was a place that offered 30 minute massages for $35, and I could get there and back in 45 minutes for my lunch break since it was on the same block. Aida was my masseuse and sometimes this treat was just what I needed to release stress and refocus on work or something productive. It was also a chance to reconnect with my body in a good way and to give it thanks for all it was undergoing. If you have an inexpensive massage place near you, I would highly recommend it while you are going through your cancer journey. If you cannot afford this, maybe your spouse, friend, or even a roommate will give you back rubs. Ever since my pregnancies my husband still rubs my feet with Gold Bond lotion for 10 minutes every night. A foot rub can do you a world of good too! Alone or with others, you can institute a new loving ritual during this time.

BUBBLE BATHS

I have always loved bubble baths and they are free, therapeutic, and harmless. Well, actually, let me *qualify* that! During chemotherapy the doctor discouraged baths, due to bacterial infections, so do ask your doctor his or her position on this. During radiation it was okay to bathe as long as you didn't get the radiated area of your breast too hot. My radiologist suggested lukewarm water that did not cover the radiated area.

I remember really missing my baths during chemotherapy. But you can take a bath a week after your lumpectomy (before chemotherapy) and after radiation (upon approval of your doctor).

When all my treatments were finished, my husband and I took a weekend trip. We got a room with a Jacuzzi tub and I bought some freesia bubble bath. This was so very healing and relaxing. I don't know if it was the jets or God's sense of humor but I only poured in a little bubble bath and this was the best bubbles I've ever had. What a treat! It totally looked like the clouds in Heaven and it was so much fun.

You can add aromatherapy or incense and candles and just relax. You definitely deserve a break. Let all your stress soak down the drain. I'm posting some pictures for you to see this mountain of bubbles because it was unreal:

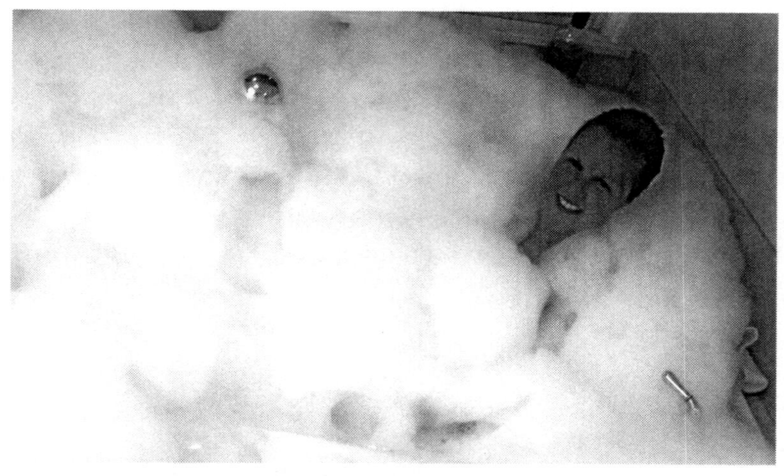

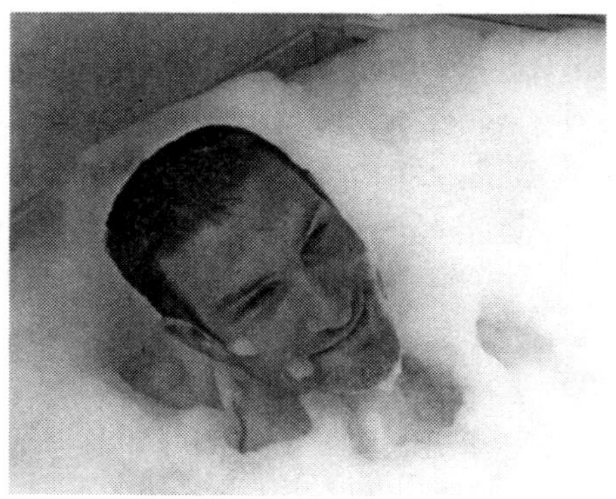

THIS IS MY HUBBY
RELAXING TOO!

This will be you. You will get to this relaxation point too at the end of your path, so just keep going!

When you can take a bath, you can also put in baking soda (without aluminum) or sea salt. This pulls out heavy metals, any radiation, and acids, and can be good for relaxation and detoxification. You can also add in grated ginger, which draws out toxins.

You can also get a natural bristle brush and brush your body in a circular motion to expel waste for two minutes each day. Skin brushing helps because your skin is the second most important channel of elimination and you want to detoxify.

CHAKRA WORK

You can work with aligning and clearing your chakras for balance. Chakras are considered wheels of energy in our body that are like data banks that record specific types of energy. Our thoughts and actions affect our chakras' functioning.

In her book, *Energy Medicine*, Donna Eden says that clearing our chakras removes toxins in our body since chakras govern the endocrine system. Bringing your chakras into balance can bring your hormones and emotions into balance. She describes how to move your hand counterclockwise over a chakra to pull out toxic energies. Afterwards you can make clockwise circles with your hand to restore the flow of energy. Check out her book *Energy Medicine* for more detailed instructions about this.

Other people clear their chakras with breathing, meditations, or chakra yoga. There are guided meditations and DVDs you can buy. See my Resource section.

Donna Eden describes chakras as energy stations where an imprint of every emotionally significant event is believed to be recorded in your chakra energy. She says that just by looking at a person's chakra energy she can know your history, obstacles to growth, your vulnerability to illness, and your soul's longings. She says that because the chakras encode experience, they often reveal how a person's history plays into their current symptoms. According to Eden, each chakra spirals down seven layers into our bodies. For her, the top layer has to do with recent events and as you go deeper, each chakra' s distinct influence becomes clear. She says the fourth level picks up early life incidents and at the fourth, fifth, and sixth levels she "sees" images and stories: at the seventh layer she sees what that person has learned in previous lifetimes. This is where the person's unfulfilled potential lies. Eden says that when she sees clear green in any of the chakras it means that healing of that chakra is underway and the energies are coming into balance.

I find it fascinating that there's a whole world of energetic healing that I have not been privy to, as a psychologist. I love to learn and now my cancer path has opened me up to more workshops and reading in a whole new field. Even though I have my Master's and Doctorate in Clinical Psychology and my coaching certification, I now see how important it can be to understand something about bodywork and energy, even if you aren't the one doing it. I cannot see chakra energy at this point (and I'm assuming most of you cannot either) but you could go see Donna Eden or practitioners like her, Anodea Judith or Carolyn Myss, or you can just learn a bit more about how your chakras work and how to clear them so they will be more balanced.

Michael Mirdad, a spiritual teacher, healer, and author who teaches the awareness of love, light, and Christ consciousness says that the seven major initiations we all experience in life relate to one or more of these centers because each chakra represents a different state of consciousness relevant to our journey toward wholeness.

I will give you a brief map of the chakras below but since there are slight variations on how the chakras are explained, take this as a generalized roadmap to these centers.

THE CHAKRA MAP

ROOT CHAKRA: this is the center of security, basic needs, finances and groundedness. It is located at the end of your spine, near your tailbone. Feel red light and safety in your root chakra and release anything that isn't pure red color.

Breathe in the rich ruby red energy and feel your roots deep in the earth as you inhale. This is a great place to connect to Mother Earth.

2nd CHAKRA: This is the center of your sexuality, creativity and your need to control. It is found at the center of your abdomen just below the navel, about two to three inches below the bellybutton. Here we hold issues of our capacity to be nurtured and our wish to be nurtured. This is the area of our occupation and creativity. It is also the area of our honor and honesty. Some say it's where the soul embraces the body and it's governed by faith and trust. Breathe in orange light into every cell.

Release anything smoky-colored and breathe in perfect orange trust from Source and creativity.

3rd CHAKRA: This is the center of power and self-esteem. It is located by your bellybutton- below your breastbone and slightly to the left. Here we record all criticism. This chakra is the center of boundaries, the sense of personal dignity and intuition. It also houses our fears and ego-needs. It is also the seat of our individual identity and ego. It houses our parental expectations. It is often logical, suspicious, and responsibility-bound, according to Donna Eden.

Breathe in the yellow power and light of God and be aware of any information about your power center. See if there is anything smoky-colored here and release it. Christopher Dilts advises we say, "What is good for God is good for me. What is good for me is good for God. Same, same." Feel God's power like the sun flowing into you so your body and creativity has this power. Christopher adds, "When the 3rd chakra is balanced you can sit like a lotus in the muck and be happy no matter what goes on around you."

4th CHAKRA: This is our Center of Self-Love and Unconditional Love. It is located in the middle of your breastbone and above the chest. It is our heart and emotions that carries our electromagnetic energy, according to Carolyn Myss, and we need them engaged to create anything. Your fourth chakra reflects how you feel about things. How is it that you love? What is your motivation? Do you love for security, comfort, money or is it about the other person? How conditional or agenda-driven is your love of yourself and others? This is also the place of forgiveness, which is important for your flow of love and energy and health.

Breathe into the heart light green energy that receives the good of God and the pure unconditional love. As you breathe out, release any unfulfilled wishes for love or any places you want to be filled. Just let them rest. Divine Mother will love them. Free your heart from desires and expectations of love from others. Your heart opens more for the good love of angels and your cup is filled to overflowing in the heart. The heart is divinely designed by God to radiate love! Communicate from fullness and overflowing instead of wants and expectations here.

5th CHAKRA: The Throat chakra is the color blue and this is the seat of your voice. It is located in your throat area. The throat chakra holds information from all your other chakras and becomes your unique expression in the world, according to Eden. No matter what the world has to say, you can speak your truth. May all you speak be of loving wisdom and kindness.

Breathe in the blue energy of your throat chakra. As you breathe out, release any stuck energy.

6th CHAKRA: This intuitive center is indigo. This is your third eye. It is located between your eyes in the middle of your forehead. It is here that you see symbols, meaning and guidance. Know your life purpose here and remember it no matter what. Connect with your vision and align your energies. Tune out the static of wants and desires that can preoccupy you and feel how peaceful it is when you are resting in your own Source and centeredness. Release any negative cording from you to others and from others to you and release lower perceptions and breathe in higher perception.

Breathe in the indigo energy into your third eye. As you breathe out, release any stuck energy. Donna Eden suggests that if you place your middle finger at the bridge of your nose and push up a couple of inches and breathe deeply, imagining that you are opening an eyelid. This technique will open your third eye.

7th CHAKRA: This crown chakra is violet and represents divine wisdom and our connection to Spirit. It is located at the top of your head. Its colors can be purple, and gold as well.

Breathe in the violet energy to receive Divine wisdom. As you breathe out, release any blocks to this chakra.

Donna Eden says that prayer, ritual, and meditation open this crown chakra.

Authors and healers who do a great job describing the chakras are Sonia Choquette, Donna Eden, Carolyn Myss, Christopher Dilts, and Anodea Judith. I've listed their books in the Resource section so that you can attend their workshops, read their books, and to learn more. I would recommend Carolyn Myss's *Energy Anatomy*, Anodea Judith's *Wheels of Light* (and her other books) and workshops with Donna Eden.

YOUR FOUNDATIONAL FIRST CHAKRA

I wanted to dedicate more time to the first chakra or the Root Chakra since it is a focus for me on my Cancer Path. For others, it may be your Heart chakra or another energy center. They say that cancer is often due to imbalances in your third and fourth chakras but I felt like my main imbalance was in my first chakra.

Our first chakra represents our personal safety, survival and foundation. It is our tribal level of knowing and it's where we first learn about our basic needs. It also governs the immune system, according to Sonia Choquette.

If you are a worrier, if you rush around a lot, ignore your body, if you have money struggles, are preoccupied with food, don't take care of yourself adequately, or feel ungrounded, then this chakra is probably imbalanced.

Your root chakra is affected by what you eat and it's good to eat food with life force like fresh fruits and vegetables to strengthen it. According to Sonia Choquette it's also affected by psychic freedom and the ability to be you. She suggests keeping plants and animals, anything alive in your home. It's also helpful to begin to take 100% responsibility for yourself and to practice impeccable self-care.

In *Energy Anatomy*, Carolyn Myss describes our root chakra as our tribal database. She says that early on our family gave us certain mores and beliefs that we bought into life about logic and the way things should be. This is our group/tribal energy and we often feel that there is safety and power in numbers. In time we need to evolve past our tribal energy into individuals but she says this tribal energy can remain strong and unconscious.

Myss also says our immune system is located in this chakra as well as any victim consciousness we may have. She says there is a reason that the AIDS consciousness spread to countries and groups who feel victimized because they lose cellular power with those thoughts and group karma. She says that if your energy is invested in tribal group systems then you can only heal at the rate at which that group is healing. Therefore, the more we plug into tribal authorities the more that determines the rate at which divine guidance comes to us and the rate at which we will heal.

She suggests we look at whether we expect society to take care of us and whether we blame people for things. She says that tribal energy is meant to keep us safe but it does not help us develop into individuals, which needs to happen. So ask yourself where you can unplug from group beliefs, expectations, and consciousness that is not healing or true for you! This is very important.

In *Energy Medicine*, Donna Eden says our first chakra grounds us and is basic to the survival of a body. It's where we store ancestral memories and trauma, going back many generations. She points out that even if traumatic experiences were faced by your parents and grandparents (and not you) their emotional imprint may still be coded in your energies. She told an interesting story where she touched a client's root chakra and knew that she might find disease in her body yet each of her chakras appeared healthy. Deeper in her root chakra she felt a terror that death was imminent. But this terror came from past generations of women who were dying in childbirth and starving. Her root chakra said, "No one can save me!" This interfered with her sense of safety and groundedness, so this energy needed to be released.

I am retelling Eden's story here because I relate to it as the child of a Holocaust survivor. I definitely had a sense of "time is running out" that doesn't seem to come from my own life experience. It is hard enough to be aware of how we encode our own life experience, much less ancestral trauma or past life experiences but it interests me that they may affect our body and healing capacity as well. Until we have reached that level of awareness, we have the option of going to healers who can help us in that domain. If you choose to do so, I urge you to go to someone who has a great reputation as a healer, or even better a practitioner recommended by reliable sources.

You can also work on healing your own root chakra by releasing any limiting tribal energy, grounding yourself through diet, structure, resources and supports, safety, addressing your finances, basic self-care and developing the freedom and space to be the real you in your life, full out! Also, connecting to Mother Earth seems especially healing for this chakra's balance and she loves you no matter what.

Christopher Dilts says that our root chakra is our connection to Mother Earth and our ability to be unconditionally loved and supported. If you felt that you never got that, you may need to learn how to parent yourself now and to free your flow of energy in your root chakra.

For myself, I needed to learn how to improve my basic self-care around food, sleep, relaxation and self-love. I wanted to pay more attention to money too so that I could provide more safety and comfort for myself and my family.

The root chakra is also the survival chakra, the place that holds our worthiness of existing. I will tell you that no matter what, you are here for a reason and you are a blessing we need on this planet! Please work to get to the place where both you and your body know this.

It is important you look at your deservingness, groundedness, and levels of support, especially when you are sick, which rocks your foundation even more.

How can you strengthen your first chakra so your foundation is stronger than ever?

Being in Nature

Look deep into nature,
and then you will understand everything better.

ALBERT EINSTEIN

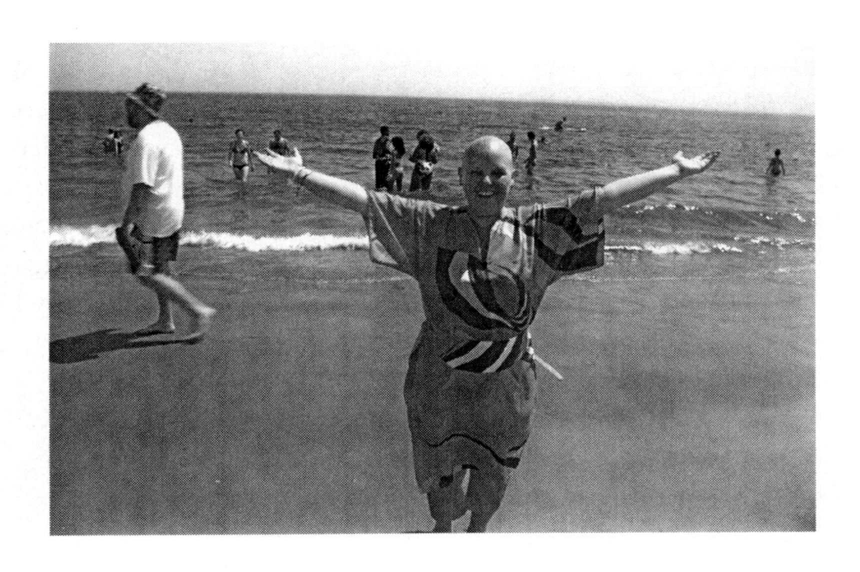

When you are doing chemotherapy and radiation you should avoid too much sun, but otherwise, being in nature is great and very healing.

Nature can also provide us with higher wisdom in many ways. I once met a fellow Beyond Words author at a media training. Her name was Catriona MacGregor. I liked her very much when we spoke briefly, and she generously gave me a copy of her book *Partnering with Nature*. It was very helpful to me after contracting breast cancer, so I'd like to share her many helpful insights about nature here. Catriona discusses how we are cut off from nature and from the animals and plants. She says that the very root of our identity is the earth. Our ancestors knew that they were one with the animals and seasons and they received great insights from the Earth. She says that the Earth generates invisible frequencies that affect us. Both the earth and our body radiate isoelectric fields, and when we align with them, we feel more balanced. Catriona says that plants continue the production of oxygen, which ensures our survival. Humans are 65% oxygen and the more oxygenated we are, the more healthy. Medical studies have shown that the more oxygenated our cells are, the less likely we are to get cancer. Catriona writes that in 1966, Otto Warbug asserted that cancer was the replacement of the respiration of oxygen in normal body cells by a fermentation of sugar. Warburg studied the impact of oxygen depletion on cells and found that when he grew animal cells under reduced oxygen pressure, that within as little as 48 hours they became cancerous. Cells taken from the same sources that were exposed to higher levels of oxygen remained healthy. Further research has since shown that cancer cells thrive in an oxygen-depleted environment and are repealed by highly oxygenated states. (Breathwork and physical activity achieve this as well).

Catriona points out that plants have long healed us and that over 100 pharmaceuticals are derived from plants. She suggests bringing plants into your home, especially if you live in the city. She points out that the alpha state we can achieve through meditation induces deep relaxation and it is the same frequency as the Earth song, which is called the Schumann resonance (at 7.83 Hertz). This may be why people feel deep peace and relaxation in meditation. She asserts that the Alpha state is the best for mind/body/spirit integration because alpha waves engage both sides of the brain instead of being confined to one area. Catriona says that spending a lot of time in beta mind states (or in logical analytic states) we starve ourselves of oxygen. Again, I would recommend reading her book to learn more about how to attune yourself to the healing frequencies of nature and Mother Earth.

Psychic John Holland says that green plants emanate prana and aliveness, which affects your aura. He also says that the ocean and its salt water has negative ions that cleanse and revitalize your aura.

We forget that we are more than just matter. We are also energetic beings. Holland says that if you can't be by the ocean you can take a salt bath instead.

In *Partnering with Nature* Catriona MacGregor says that negative ions are easily inhaled into the lungs and absorbed into the bloodstream. They have been found to alleviate depression and stress and to boost energy. They increase your serotonin, raise your spirits, and accelerate the delivery of oxygen to your cells. Who might have thought that nature was energetic medicine?

Find a park or body of water near you and visit it regularly while you are going through treatment. Listen to the messages you receive.

Deep Breathing

I took a deep breath and listened to the old bray of my heart.
I am. I am. I am.

Sylvia Path

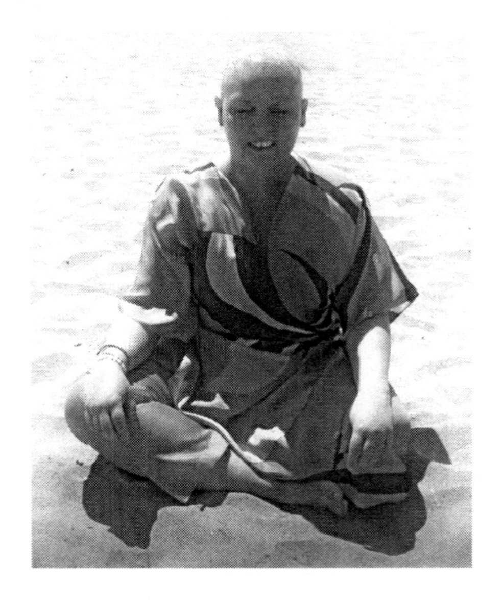

My mentor Christopher Dilts makes a really big deal about breathing. He says that the great masters all say, "Quality of breath equals quality of mind." He says that deep breathing relaxes you and engages your parasympathetic nervous system so that you can heal. When you are stressed and very busy (like me) you often talk fast and breathe shallowly, and this activates your sympathetic nervous system in a "fight or flight" mode. Cancer thrives in this environment. So, if you practice deep breathing you can put your body back into a restorative mode and oxygenate your organs pretty easily. Christopher Dilts likes to joke that "We all have time to breathe because you have to breathe anyway!"

I also read that deep breathing is helpful to your lymphatic system, which protects your body from infection and disease via your immune response. It boosts your level of oxygen and nutrients as well.

In *Energy Medicine*, Donna Eden also suggests that breathing can be helpful for pain. She likens this to how a Lamaze breathing helps women through labor, and recommends breathing through the nostrils with your mouth closed, as if smelling a rose. Then breathe out as if blowing out a candle. She says, "As you exhale, you can release some of the energy involved with the pain."

I would recommend taking 15 minutes two times a day for deep breathing. You can use some guided tapes in the Resource section if you need more structure to institute this practice. You can do it anywhere, as often as you like and there is no cost or downside. Plus, it only takes 10 minutes. I've included some CDs in my Resource section in case you want to do deep breathing with a guide.

Your Diet

Let food be thy medicine.

Hippocrates

I never thought that much about what I ate. Other than diet coke drinking, I ate like the average busy professional person who was often on the run and didn't much like to cook.

Then enter the cancer diagnosis. I asked my oncologist and surgeon at Sloan whether my diet mattered. Both of them said not to worry about it during chemotherapy. One said just to eat a balanced diet and there was nothing I couldn't eat, even soy. My doctor at Beth Israel also told me that the research showed that once you had cancer, diet didn't really affect it. I thought to myself, if that is the case, then why do so many people say the exact opposite? What is true?

This also left an impression on my husband, who was a meat and potatoes guy and who generally did all the cooking. When I suggested buying organic or juicing he'd roll his eyes and remind me that the doctors all said that diet didn't affect cancer. He thought I was making it up. This made it harder to get the foods I needed and to eliminate any tempting sugary foods from our household.

Plus, it was confusing to get so many different opinions about diet within my healing team. My doctors said it didn't matter and my husband agreed with them. After both oncologists said my diet did not matter my husband thought I was crazy for trying to make all those uncomfortable healthful changes. Dan, my neighbor and health coach recommended the Ketogenic diet that is very low carbohydrates, moderate to low protein, and high in healthy fats. Susan Silberstein a cancer health counselor from beatcancer.org recommended the opposite: a vegan-type diet with fiber, vegetables and fruits and little meat or carbohydrates. Christopher, my Spiritual mentor agreed with Susan, as did my doctor friend Ana.

Interestingly, I read that The American Cancer society estimates that diet is a primary factor in a third of cancer deaths. So, again I ask, "Which is it?"

Without giving a definitive answer, let me explore different views on diet and then I will share what I decided for myself as a patient. Maybe sorting through this weighing process with me will help you because you are bound to encounter proponents of different approaches and opinions as well and I know you want to do whatever is in your control to heal.

THE VEGAN-LIKE DIET STANCE

Many have said that cancer likes an environment of dehydration, acidic foods, stress, red meat and sugar. So, to combat cancer I should drink a lot of water, eat alkaline foods like vegetables, drink green juice and avoid carbs like white flour, bagels, pizza, breads and desserts, and induce relaxation. I had been eating acidic foods like flour, chocolate, meat, poultry, dairy, sugar, soda and tea. Susan from www.beatcancer.org concurred with my revised diet approach from a health perspective, although she allowed oatmeal, quinoa, and brown rice for carbohydrates.

I had phone sessions with Susan Silberstein and she told me that 70% of breast cancer cases are avoidable through dietary changes, according to the National Cancer Institute. She says that the cause of the cancer is often the cure and if you can repair that you can prevent recurrence. She said that in her opinion cancer patients rarely die of tumors, they die of malnutrition, toxemia and infections, and good nutrition can address all of these. According to Susan, a heavily plant-based diet, low in fat, with little or no animal protein constitutes an excellent anti-cancer diet.

She advised that I eliminate yogurt, dairy, and most meat—due to the growth hormones, which can also grow the cancer cells. Susan cited a study of nearly 26,000 women who ate meat more than five times per week and had 2.5 times greater risk for breast cancer than those who ate meat fewer than 2 times a week (International Journal of Cancer, 1995). I also watched a video on Netfix called *Forks Over Knives* where their research suggested that there was more cancer in certain parts of China where they consumed higher amounts of meat.

Vegans have been trying to get my attention for a long time now. When I lived in Pennsylvania (for graduate school) two of my dear friends were vegans. Ana was a doctor friend who taught patients how to shop and eat healthy and my friend Ann was a fellow psychologist who married a vegan and raised her daughter vegan. I saw the great effects it had on both of them and it inspired me, but I guess not enough to stick with it, especially once I moved away to New York City. The third sign was my sister Avra and her boyfriend turned mostly vegan. Seeing how healthy and happy they were was great plus all of them lost weight. Another friend, my life coach Terri, developed Crohn's disease and once she became vegan she too felt much better. So, the signs were all around me but I had chosen not to act on this path right away.

Look around and see if there are any role models for this path in your life. Has the universe been trying to get your attention? Are there new and exciting ways you can reintroduce vegetables into your life? Usually if I see something important show up in my life three times, I pay attention.

If I'm lazy and still don't love to cook but want to add veggies to my diet, I just boil water and make brussel sprouts with sea salt or broccoli or sweet peas and eat it when I'm working, accompanied by a glass of green tea. This takes all of 6 minutes, and barely counts as "cooking" in my books.

But even though I've moved towards this direction now, I still eat some meat and seafood. I'm like the guy who is careful not to give his word unless he'll commit for life. *Is this a phase?* I wonder. Will I still continue all these healthy habits after the 5 year remission window? I guess time will tell.

THE KETOGENIC DIET

There are also people who will tell you it's better to eat high fat, moderate to low in protein, and low carbs. Dan, my neighbor and health coach advocated eating a Keytogenic Diet which studies show can slow down the rate of cancer growth and development. Dan explained that you can get energy through sugar or fat but that you don't get energy from protein directly. When you eat excess protein it converts into glucose which your body uses like sugar. So moderating protein for people who eat protein is something to consider, like having less than 60 grams of protein. He says you need to decide if you are going to be a sugar burner or a fat burner, so that your body has energy to function. Dr. Craig Thompson, the President of Sloan Kettering Hospital in New York says that fat doesn't increase cancer at all, carbohydrates do dramatically, and protein falls somewhere in between.

Dan says the American Diet is high in carbohydrates and this is not good for weight loss and can contribute to insulin resistance or cancer. For example, he points out that two slices of whole wheat bread can raise your blood sugar more than a Snickers bar. He says that this chronically high blood sugar from high sugar and fructose consumption increases our risk for all modern diseases that hunter gatherers didn't have. This includes cancer, heart disorder, high blood pressure, strokes and diabetes.

Dan says that when you eat 40-60 grams of protein, for the average-sized person this won't turn into fat. It's used to create hormones, rebuild muscle tissue and body tissues. He says with vegan diets it's hard to get enough complete proteins (without the carbs) and you can be deficient in serotonin, omega 3's, dopamine and other essential hormones which can lead to risk factors for multiple neurodegenerative diseases and emotional disturbances. Dan says, "By definition, a low-fat diet is a high carb diet because of the carbohydrates."

He says that if you eat carbohydrates they are turned into sugar and insulin and then into body fat. Whereas if you eat fat directly, it's the only macronutrient that won't elicit an insulin response. He cites The Warburg Effect named after a Nobel Prize winning scientist who claimed that almost all cancers exclusively feeds on sugar and when cancer cells consume ketones they die. Dan says that ketones are energy from fat. This includes food like coconut oil, olive oil, grassfed organic butter, any animal protein, seafood or nuts.

When I told Dan I'd rather not eat meat, he recommended I eat mussels and seafood.

I have opted for veggies, some fruit, organic chicken, and seafood, which sounds similar to what Louise Hay describes as her diet. I still don't know how to fully reconcile these two stances but most people do agree that sugar and cancer are not a good combination! What Dan was trying to convey is that it makes no difference between eating savory foods like cake and candy or foods that turn into sugar like cereals, breads (whole or white), rice or starches.

THE MACROBIOTIC DIET & KRIS CARR

I attended Kris Carr's workshop at NY Omega when I was going through treatment. Kris is the author of the documentary *Crazy, Sexy*

Cancer. She was diagnosed with an incurable cancer and she changed her diet and lifestyle. Then she started teaching others what she had learned. I found her to be very inspiring and I bought several of her cookbooks, which I would also recommend. You can rent her film to learn more about her cancer journey. She calls food her Original Medicine and she believes that juicing releases toxins, so she juices a lot. She also advocates colonics and feels that the cause of disease is inflammation which includes your eating, drinking, and thinking! She agrees with most of what Susan Silberstein says dietarily, so I won't repeat all that information again here. She stresses that the raw food diet is loaded with enzymes and gives you energy. It is oxygen rich and full of nutrients.

It is notable that she allows herself whole grains like spelt, kamut, soba noodles, millet, quinoa, brown rice, buck wheat and some bread brands like Ezekiel sprouted bread and Alvarado Street Sprouted Wheat. She also suggests Lara bars, sweet potato chips and air popped popcorn as snacks. I would love to add in some of these bread products again but I get confused as to whether it will spike my insulin levels. It definitely seems like browns and wheat are better than white pastas and breads.

Carr also says that if you are not evacuating daily then there's something wrong in your diet. She suggests doing a stool, blood, saliva and urine sample once a year and tells people to keep a 10-day food journal to make yourself conscious of what you are eating. I would recommend that you take one of her workshops and read her books. She is a fellow cancer sister and walks her talk!

METABOLIC SYNDROME AND WEIGHT GAIN

There may be other dietary concerns specific for cancer patients, like Metabolic Syndrome. Metabolic Syndrome is often correlated with inflammation and risk factors like high blood glucose, high blood pressure, abdominal obesity and cholesterol problems. Women with triple-negative breast cancer are much more likely to have metabolic syndrome than women with other forms of breast cancer. I know I have 30 pounds of excess tummy fat after my second pregnancy and that can cause insulin spikes, which is not good for cancer.

My neighbor Dan gave me an article on Metabolic syndrome because I had gained weight with my second pregnancy and I still looked pregnant. I have 30 pounds to lose and it's all in my stomach area which is why Dan suspected I was on a continuum leading to Metabolic Syndrome. During my 8 months of treatment, no doctors mentioned it. Interestingly, when my mom spoke to a psychic and asked about my breast cancer, she told her it was triggered by hormones released from my second pregnancy and my weight gain. So, who knows, but it seems wise to try and lose that tummy weight!

The article Dan emailed me was called, "Weight Gain, Metabolic Syndrome, and Breast Cancer Recurrence: Are Dietary Recommendations Supported by Data?" from the *International Journal of Breast Cancer*, Volume 2012. It explains that Metabolic Syndrome can include weight gain, central obesity, elevated serum insulin and glucose and insulin resistance, which has been strongly associated with breast cancer recurrence and worst outcomes after treatment. Breast cancer patients with Metabolic Syndrome undergoing chemotherapy were found to have an overall poor response to treatment, and those with specifically high blood glucose levels had more disease progression. As a principal energy source of cancer cells, elevated glucose may fuel tumor progression.

In one study, women in the highest quartile of insulin had a two-fold risk of tumor recurrence and a three-fold increase in risk of death versus patients in the lowest quartile.

Metformin (a drug often used for diabetics) sensitizes patients to lower circulating glucose and insulin levels, and is being considered for use in breast cancer patients with the aggressive type of cancer that I have (triple negative breast cancer). So it appears that insulin and sugar may fuel cancer cells. More bad news! I love sugar, and maybe you do too.

Current diet strategies for breast cancer employ low-fat diets with increased fruit intake, grains, and vegetables as carbohydrate sources, but some studies show that patients tend to gain weight. All these foods turn to sugar and if sugars feed cancers this may not be good. Weight gain after breast cancer treatment has a poor prognosis and may raise recurrence. Animal studies show that after a breast cancer diagnosis, between 50-96% of patients gain weight. Perhaps it's also due to stress.

Dan's point in sending me this article was to remind me that it's important not to eat too many carbohydrates or sugar with my type of cancer.

Of course reading this research made me thankful that people like Susan and Dan alerted me to the importance of diet early on since my doctors had minimized it. Was this your experience too? As patients we want to empower ourselves to be agents in our healing and diet is one thing we can do towards that end.

Letting go of sugars and carbohydrates has not been an easy shift for me. Recent studies have shown that sugar is more addictive than crack or cocaine, so it may be hard for us to successfully decrease carbohydrates in the middle of such a stressful treatment and time period, but we should at least have the information and understanding to make this gradual shift.

So, be honest with yourself about your dietary habits, discuss diet with your doctor, and do an inventory of sugar and insulin in your diet. Find new sources of sweetness elsewhere (see my chapter on joy) so you can minimize recurrence. Having said that, even with the best intentions, it's not always easy and I still have a ways to go with this myself!

Again, I am not a nutritionist. I'm just including this section as a patient, to show how confusing the information on diet can be. You will encounter many well-meaning, intelligent professionals along your path who will say different things, and no doubt compelling research for each position! You may prefer to automatically defer to your doctor on every matter, but I felt that would be a mistake for me. After all, if what we eat matters in a regular, healthy lifestyle, so should it matter even more when you are unwell.

GET HELP COOKING

As I said, I don't like to cook and had little time to do so, so I decided to get some help. My mom drafted my neighbor Dan (who has a company called Workaholic Workouts) to help me with my diet, cooking, and exercise. He gave her a discounted rate as my next door neighbor and he was close at hand, which was very helpful. The great thing about Dan is that when I explained my original plan was not to eat too much meat, he listened and supported me, even though that was not his usual food philosophy. He even started cooking some meals for me and would drop them off, which was a huge help. Salads had apple, nuts, spices, and cranberries—and tasted great! I will put Dan's information in the appendix of this book so you can contact him (or someone like him if you live elsewhere) to help you. Take it from me, you are much more likely to eat foods that are good for you if they taste good and are convenient. It also helps to have someone to check in with you and encourage you.

MY FOOD CHANGES

I don't know if I made the best decisions but these are the food changes I made. I eliminated dairy from my diet due to the growth hormones and casein. I drank almond, rice, and coconut milk instead. I continued eating eggs and ate So Delicious coconut milk yogurt. I ate very little cheese and tried to eat organic cheese when I did.

I eliminated red meat and just had a little chicken, fish, mussels and shrimp. Susan Silberstein of beatcancer.org says that fat promotes a hormone called estradol, which decreases on a low fat diet. She says that high fat diets also promote storage of xenoestrogens which love fatty tissue and store dangerous compounds. Animal protein diets are very acidic which creates mucus in the body and can clog your elimination. Also, cancer thrives in acidic environments. Researchers who studied 61,000 women showed that the consumption of fat boosted the breast cancer risk 69%. She says that high animal protein raises prolactin which can stimulate breast cancer as well as growth hormones. One study showed a 25% increased risk in breast cancer with red meat consumption. When Japanese women began to eat meat daily, they developed a 6 times higher risk of breast cancer than those who never eat meat. Also, the more well-cooked your meat, the more carcinogens, which can damage your DNA by emitting radioactivity.

I thought chicken was better. But authors of *The Complete Cancer Cleanse* point out that when chicken is cooked it produces heterocyclic amines (HCAs) which are the same carcinogens as in tobacco smoke. HCAs are 15 times more concentrated in grilled chicken than in beef. Also, one-third of packaged chicken in supermarkets has live salmonella bacteria inside the plastic. So if you choose to eat meat anyway, buy organic and bake it, but definitely don't char it.

I ate more vegetables and tried to get green juices at least twice a week. According to Susan Silberstein, juicing provides the body with concentrated phytonutrients, enzymes, minerals, caretenoids and anti-oxidants. This cleanses the liver, neutralizes cancer causing free radicals and enhances immune function. It creates an alkaline environment which remedies acidosis, on which cancer cells thrive. Susan says that the best combinations of juice are organic carrot, carrot-spinach, carrot-kale, carrot-beet and cucumber juices. She suggests getting a Champion juicer and says that you can store juices in your refrigerator for up to 12 hours. Susan does not see a problem with juicing during chemotherapy and radiation, since it's just proper nutrition. My doctors said not to juice during chemotherapy, so for the most part I waited until after chemotherapy to boost my immune system. This is another area of discrepancy.

I cut out most carbs, occasionally allowing myself Ezekiel bread, oatmeal, Smart Bran cereal, quinoa and rice. Carbs like white sugar and flour increase insulin and can promote cell growth. My neighbor Dan pointed out that carbs are not always what they seem so it's good to check the label for the number of carbs. For example, he looked up brown rice (which people think is healthier) and showed me that brown rice had 140 carbs in one cup, while white rice had only 53 carbs. Ezekiel cereal (which I thought was especially healthy) had 32 carbs but Smart Bran cereal has less.

He also gave me an article on carbohydrate restriction in the treatment and prevention of cancer by Klement and Kamnerer (2011). The article suggests that by systematically reducing the amount of dietary carbs you consume, you can suppress or at least delay the emergence of cancer and the proliferation of already existing tumor cells can be slowed down. Glucose can have direct and indirect effects on tumor cell proliferation: most malignant cells depend on steady glucose availability of fatty acid or ketone bodies due to mitochondrial dysfunction. Also, high insulin-like growth factor (IGF-1) levels can promote cell proliferation via the insulin IGF-1 signaling pathways. A number of mouse models have shown anti-tumorigenic properties of very low ketogenic diets.

I eliminated most sugar because one thing that doctors and nutritionists agree on is that *it feeds the cancer cells.* I started using Truvia or Stevia in my drinks: a low glycemic diet may lower your risk of getting cancer by 253%. Cells need oxygen to metabolize minerals and vitamins to thrive. When cells cannot use oxygen to metabolize, they resort to fermenting glucose for their energy. In a study by Dr. Colin Chemp, he says that even one meal (one time) where a patients eats carbohydrates can make their blood sugar go over 180 and can shorten their lives by 8 months!

I tried (and often failed) to drink 8 bottles of essential water (which is supposed to be alkaline and has a 9.5 pH level). Sometimes I drank green tea, iced green tea with ginger, coconut milk, unsweetened ice tea with Stevia or water with lemon, elderberry extract and Stevia. You would think that drinking water would be simple but not for me! My dad took a bunch of bottles of water into the city and lined them up on my window sill in my psychotherapy office. I truly believe that experiencing how difficult it is to make changes will help me to be a more compassionate healer. Shifting a number of ingrained habits at once when you are busy is tough.

I also eliminated alcohol which elevates serum estrogen levels, especially estradiol. One study showed that women who drink one alcoholic drink a day were 39% more likely to develop breast cancer than those who did not drink. A study in the *Journal of Oncology* found survivors who have one or more drinks a day have a 90% risk of recurrence.

I decreased diet soda which causes acid. Caffeine also isn't good for cancer because caffeine promotes breast dysplasia and cell change towards malignancy. Caffeine is found in coffee, tea, soda, chocolate, peanuts and cheese. In *Knockout*, Dr. Burzynski says that soda can silence a number of genes, which is scary.

I tried to watch the fats I ate because Omega 3 oils are much better than Omega 6 fats. Omega 3 fats decrease inflammation. Researchers who studied 61,000 women found that regular consumption of Omega 6 fats increased breast cancer 69%. Omega 6 fats to avoid included sunflower oil, safflower oil, soybean oil, corn oil, sesame oil and peanut oil. Better Omega 3 fats include fish, eggs, walnuts, pumpkin seeds and flaxseeds. Omega 3, found in olive oil and coconut oil, keeps cell membranes elastic, allowing oxygenation and healthy cell functioning. I bought coconut oil from Trader Joes when I needed to cook something with oil, or else I used olive oil.

Foods that I tried to add more of were vegetables, salmon, lentils, kidney beans, some fruits (2 a day), green tea, eggs, almond butter, almond milk, green vegetable juice, oatmeal and tumeric powder.

Susan Silberstein also suggested adding flaxseed, raw walnuts, pumpkin seeds, olive oil, pomegranates, beets, watermelon, broccoli, Brussels sprouts, and bok choy.

I invite you to explore your diet for yourself so that you can feel as healthy as possible. I do intuitively believe that diet affects health and I did not delve into the contradictory research on diets too much, but I urge you to become informed and decide what works best for your body type. Remember that you can also use Donna Eden's suggestion to energy test the food for your body type.

I bought Kris Carr's book, *Crazy Sexy Kitchen: 150 Plant-Empowered Recipes to Ignite a Mouthwatering Revolution*, and actually started to cook a little.

Here's some additional information I found about how particular foods may affect cancer.

Flaxseeds

Flaxseeds bind estrogen and improve bowel function. Flaxseeds reduce your cancer risk 54% according to some studies. Susan suggests using 2 tablespoons of freshly ground flaxseed in oatmeal, sprinkled on salads or in juices. I bought ground flaxseed and was told by my neighbor that it gets rancid right away so you need to be sure to keep it refrigerated.

Green Tea

Green tea has antioxidant compounds that fight cancer. In one study the cancer survivors given green tea were 94% higher than the non-tea cancer survivor rate, which was 33%.

Shitake Mushrooms

Shitake mushrooms contain lentinen, which increases cell counts to combat cancer.

Lentils & Legumes

Lentils are great protein. You can easily and cheaply eat them too.

I recommend Amy's lentil soup or Amy's black bean soup in cans. Legumes include lentils, black peas, peas and soybeans. They deliver saponins, protease inhibitors and phytic acid, which remove toxins and build cells.

Cabbage

According to Jennifer Grifin in her oprah.com article,"11 Tips to Get Through Chemotherapy," cancer hates cabbage—so eat up, girls!

Chia Seeds

These are good to put on your oatmeal, in salads or in vegetable stir fries. They have Omega 3.

Ginger

This is great for anti-nausea. I got ginger candies for nausea and would go to Argo Tea twice a week on my way to the office to get a large iced ginger tea with an extra shot of ginger. This was heavenly and replaced my diet coke habit. You can also make it at home. Regular ginger also has been said to induce cancer cell death.

Garlic

Garlic is a cancer suppressing agent, according to authors of *The Complete Cancer Cleanse.* It detoxifies heavy metals in the body and toxins. Dr. Benjamin Lau says that garlic nullifies the effects of radiation. The garlic' s antimicrobial properties come from an enzyme called *allacin*, which is freed after the garlic is cut or chopped. You can chop garlic and eat it raw, or chop it and let it sit 15 minutes before you cook it. If you just cook it whole it won't have those anti-cancer properties.

Parsley

Parsley protects against carcinogens and regulates the body's production of prostaglandin, a substance that promotes tumors, according to Sharie Calbom in *The Complete Cancer Cleanse.*

Onions

Onions are a source of flavonoid quercitin, which has been shown to inhibit proliferation of human breast cancer cells in test tubes and it's good for liver detoxification.

Curcumin

My neighbor and health coach Dan sent me an important article that I've referenced in the Resource section. My breast cancer was triple negative, which means the cells don't have the characteristic receptors for estrogen, progesterone and HER2/neu, so it's considered most resistant because these missing receptors are required for many conventional treatments. Fifteen to twenty-five percent of all breast cancers are triple negative like mine. A new study from China indicates that a compound in turmeric, known as *curcumin*, is capable of inducing programmed cell death within triple negative breast cancer cells! Greenmedinfo.com has indexed over 60 in vitro and animal studies demonstrating curcumin's anti-breast cancer activity, or its ability to enhance chemotherapy treatment. Dan says that if you add black pepper to it, you make it 10,000 percent more bio available. So, why don't you spice up your stir-fry and vegetable drinks with tumeric and some pepper?

Veggies

According to Harvard researchers, women who eat two plus servings of cartenoid rich fruits and veggies have a 17% lower risk for breast cancer. Cruciferous vegetables include broccoli, cabbage, cauliflower, chard, and kale to help regulate body enzymes that defend against cancer.

Pomegranate

Pomegranate may reduce cancer up to 87% according to one recent study.

Broccoli

Some studies say that broccoli kills cancer cells, so add this to meals.

Authors of *The Complete Cancer Cleanse* say that within hours of broccoli's arrival in the stomach, carcinogens leave the cells. Plus, it's yummy!

Red Fruits & Vegetables

Tomatoes, pink grapefruit, and watermelon have *lycopene*, which protects cells from free radicals. Berries are great sources of Vitamin C and have phytochemicals that are anti-cancer agents. Strawberries and raspberries contain *ellagic acid*, which is an antioxidant that slows reproduction of cancer cells. Be sure your oncologist allows you to eat berries during chemotherapy—most will.

THE BUDWIG DIET

A German biochemist called Joanne Budwig discovered that if you combine cottage cheese with flaxseed oil this would increase oxygen supply to your cells, and cancer doesn't like oxygen.

So try taking 2/3 of a cup of cottage cheese with 6 tablespoons of flaxseed oil and you can mix in some berries with it in a blender. Eat this once a day, taken in two doses. This reportedly gets to the cell membrane, increasing the oxygen to the cell membrane and increasing the cellular energy production. See also http://www.budwigcenter.com/anti-cancer-diet.php.

ABSORBING CHANGES SLOWLY

I know this healthy diet sounds gross, but you get used to it, especially if you feel your life is at stake. Most doctors agree that excess weight around your belly area isn't good for cancer due to insulin production. So, hopefully this plant-based diet will help me lose weight *and* become healthier.

When I first started to make dietary changes, I avoided going to big family parties with tons of pies and food. I was going through treatment, I was tired, and I needed to really consolidate my diet without public pressure and opinion. Later, when I attended such events I would just bring my own food. It wasn't that hard. So if you do make such big dietary changes, give yourself a learning curve and some time. If you have a bad day during chemo and need some comfort food, don't beat yourself up. Just try and get back on the horse because you, your health, and your body are worth it!

Remember that making so many changes at once can be a challenge. Be compassionate with yourself. Sometimes you'll take two steps forward and one step back. Also, try and think of some sweet things you can eat as a reward on occasion, like baked apple or fruit sorbet or Quest bars in brownie flavor. I will add some information about Quest bars in the Resource section. They are yummy and are low in sugar content compared to many protein bars.

Just accepting that you have cancer is hard enough, and then giving up all your favorite comfort foods like sugar, carbs, soda, baked goods, soda and alcohol, and even most meat doesn't seem fair. Training yourself is somewhat like training a dog. It takes constant repetition and no compromise. Visualize yourself drinking 8 glasses of water, breathing and resting, and then you can do it in baby steps. Really you can!

THE MICROWAVE

Another big shift in our house was that Susan told me that I should give up the microwave. In all my rushing around and dislike of cooking I didn't realize that I used it a lot. I'd use it to make tea, warm up food the nanny made, or to cook frozen food. Even though intellectually I knew I shouldn't use the microwave, it was convenient. Plus, from the brief Internet search I did, reviews and research about microwave use were mixed as well.

Some said that *microwaving did not cause cancer* because the microwave was non-ionizing radiation and it is ionizing radiation that can cause it. Ionizing radiation can damage any cell in the body. But it all depends on how much radiation the cell gets. Ionizing radiation is made of high-energy waves and the energy can get into cells and chemically change the way the cell works. This process is called ionization. Very small amounts of ionizing radiation don't do much harm but too much can cause burns, radiation sickness, and cancer. The genetic material of a cell (known as DNA) is very sensitive to ionizing radiation. DNA is a code for all the genes that carry the instructions for how our body works and its characteristics, and Ionizing radiation can change a cell's DNA. It is then possible for the cell to do something very different from what it is supposed to do, like become cancerous and keep reproducing in an uncontrolled way. This could take years but cancer may eventually develop. There are 3 main types of ionizing radiation including Natural background radiation, Medical Radiation, and Non-Medical Radiation.

Natural background radiation comes from radioactive substances in the soil, Radioactive gases given off from the earth, such as radon, very small amounts of radioactivity in the body and cosmic rays from the solar system (the sun, stars and outer space). **Medical radiation** includes diagnostic radiology, like X-ray machines, nuclear medicine, like drinking a radioactive substance to diagnose or treat diseases and radiotherapy, which uses high energy rays to kill cancer cells. **Non-medical radiation** includes nuclear radiation that comes from previous nuclear weapon explosions or accidents throughout the world, like in Chernobyl.

Proponents for microwaving say that non-ionizing radiation has enough energy to move things around inside a cell but not enough to change cells chemically. They say that the only type of non-ionizing radiation that we know can cause cancer is over exposure to ultraviolet rays, which causes skin cancer.

Microwaves do produce a magnetic field while they are in use. This drops sharply the further you are from the oven, and doesn't last long.

Those against microwaving say that *microwaving does cause cancer.* Hans Hertel, a Swiss researcher, links cancer to microwave cooking, explaining that normally cooked food is heated from the outside in: microwave radiation heats from the inside out. Hertel explains that technically produced microwaves alternate current. Atoms, molecules and cells hit by this hard electromagnetic radiation are forced to reverse polarity 1 to 100 billion times a second. No atoms, molecules or cells of any organic system can withstand such a violent, destructive power for any extended period of time, not even in the low energy range of milliwatts. Structures of molecules are torn apart, molecules are deformed and become impaired in quality.

Besides these thermal modifications, there is also direct damage to cell walls and genes from microwaves. The cells are actually broken, neutralizing the electrical potentials between the outer and inner sides of the cell membranes, according to Hertel.

Strange and unknown compounds are created by microwave energy's penetration into organic matter. They are called *radiolytic* compounds. Hertel's research has indicated that *far more radiolytic compounds are created by microwave cooking than regular cooking.*

Hertel concludes that the food damaged from microwaving modifies the cellular activity in the human consumers of that food. One`s cells are forced by the damaged cells and radiolytic compounds to adapt into an emergency mode of energy production. The human cells are forced from normal cellular oxidation into the anaerobic energy production of glucose fermentation, which is a cancerous condition.

According to Hertel, anaerobic glucose fermentation is how cancer cells survive and thrive. This is why cancer cells cannot exist in oxygen. This is why cancer patients should not eat sugar or foods made with sugar.

I'm not a scientist, and as a breast cancer patient I'm not entirely sure what is true or what future research will show. To err on the safe side, try not to use your microwave as much or at all. Pretend you're from an earlier, simpler time and see how that goes or just hide it away for awhile.

RAW FOODS

Many people say that raw foods are especially good for you because of the sunlight they contain and the vital energy. Author Sonia Choquette says that spiritual people normally gravitate to foods that hold more sunlight and energy, so eating these foods may even hold a spiritual benefit. When my sister and her boyfriend Albert visited they were good role models because they eat mostly raw foods. They made big salads, and ate lots of fruit, nuts, and seeds. They looked so happy and relaxed, and made eating fun. So, I always think of them as good role models for this lifestyle, as well as my friend Ana. She used to host healthy food parties in Pennsylvania. I have a picture of my sister and Albert eating a beautiful salad above my desk to remind me to eat well.

Most of us weren't raised to eat such healthy food and we have many role models of the opposite. You may even experience well-meaning peer pressure to try the pie, or meatloaf, in your social settings. For this reason, it's important to surround yourself with supportive people who understand your healthy path, and can teach you new ways to make changing your eating habits fun and show you the benefits. You can go to a raw foods class or bond with other cancer survivors who are eating this way. Put out the intention and you will find some support.

It's also best to buy organic fruits and vegetables if you can. A four-year European Union-funded study found that organic fruits and vegetables contain up to 40 percent more ant-oxidants. If you can't afford to go all organic then look at the "Dirty Dozen" list which annually rates fruits and vegetables from worst to best at www.ewg.org. You can cut pesticide exposure 90 percent by avoiding the 12 conventionally grown fruits and veggies found to be most contaminated. Briefly, the foods most important to buy organic are peaches, apples, sweet bell peppers, celery, nectarines, strawberries, cherries, kale, lettuce, grapes, carrots and pears; but check the most current list.

WATER

This may sound strange (because water is essentially tasteless) but I was never a fan of water. I needed to drink 8 bottles of water a day to flush out the chemo chemicals so I would try and number the bottles to keep track. See the pic:

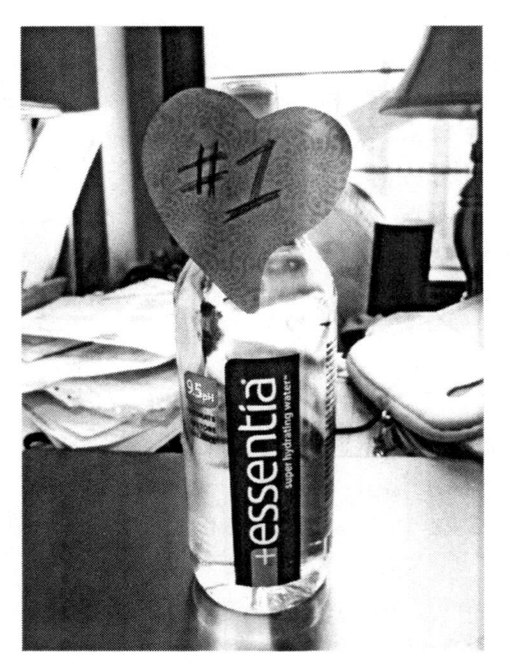

The truth is I never drank eight bottles a day consistently, but if you dislike water this numbering system may at least keep you honest. My dad ordered me two cases of Essentia water every month because we heard it is the most alkaline water. Another one that's easier to get in delis is Fiji water. By the way, after forcing myself to drink water

I started to find it refreshing so you might too. I flavored my water bottles with lemon juice, Stevia, or Elderberry sometimes. Stevia actually helps regulate blood sugar levels and it doesn't cause the pancreas to produce excess insulin. Plus, most other artificial sugars are even worse than sugar. So try it out!

Water helps kidneys flush excess acid and gets out toxins. Donna Eden also adds, "Water conducts electricity and dehydration interferes with the flow of energy in your body." So, drinking water facilitates energy production and also keeps our lymphatic system clean.

GREEN JUICE

Christopher Dilts told me the website fountainofyouthjuices.com has recipes for making your own juices, or you can call the owner Abdulah for help. Also, Kris Carr, author of *Crazy, Sexy Cancer* has a website www.crazyjuice.com that has 60 juicing recipes. Many people carry green powder with them instead of making fresh vegetable juice when they travel. there are many good ones on the market. This could also be a convenience option for you if you aren't hands-on in the kitchen.

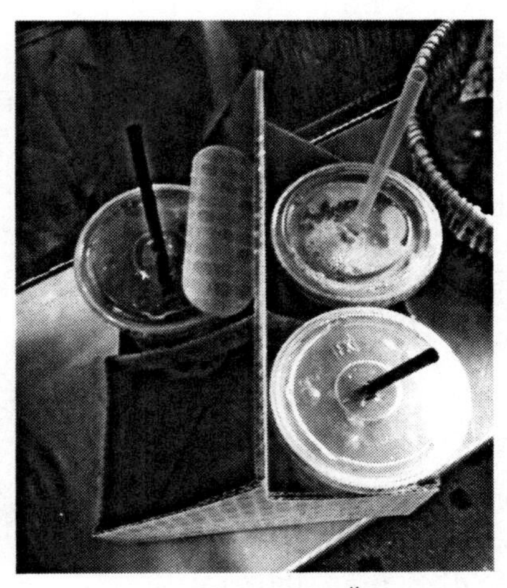

THIS WAS JUICE #33 THAT I WOULD GET RIGHT NEAR MY OFFICE

What I've done for convenience and to introduce green juices into my lifestyle is to order Green Juice (made by Blueprint) from Fresh Direct. It's about $10 for a large bottle and I can grab it and take it to work. I usually order 2 a week. I also found a vendor near my office who makes fresh vegetable juices for $5 so I grab that on the way to work two days a week: he has

4 locations around NYC. Many health food stores make fresh juice as well, so if you look I am sure you will find something near you, or you can buy a juicer and do it yourself. Some recommended brands of juicers include Champion.

A popular green juice recipe is kale, spinach, cucumber, avocado, carrot and an apple, if you want to make it yourself. Some recommend adding liquid Stevia French vanilla (instead of sugar) to make any leafy green mixture sweeter. I had a blender called The Healthmaster by Montel Williams before my husband got me a juicer for Hanukkah. I would make vegetable smoothies in the morning with almond milk, half a banana, 1 tablespoon almond butter, half a cucumber and handfuls of frozen kale, broccoli and spinach. I'd put a few drops of liquid Stevia in and it would taste delicious! His website, www.myhealthmaster.com, also has lots of good recipes. I've also listed two juicing books in the bibliography that may be helpful.

Sure, it's easier to grab a bacon, egg and cheese on a roll on your way to work, but what I just described is not that hard to make and it is so good for you. This is just about creating new habits that are full of self-love.

Carrot juicing has powerful cancer fighting properties. Doctors suggest drinking 2 pints a day. You can also try carrot-apple juice.

Your oncologist may say that he or she prefers you to eat cooked vegetables instead of juicing them during chemo therapy because they are concerned about bacteria and feel that cooking helps to kill them. Most alternative healers think juicing during chemotherapy is fine but you will need to talk to your doctor and decide for yourself. If you are worried, you can eat greens other ways and start juicing following your chemotherapy.

As an alternative, Susan Silberstein from also recommends capsules called Juice Plus for busy people who don't eat enough vegetables. I did not try this yet but many people use this product and love it. She recommends taking 6 fruit and veggie capsules per day with plenty of water. If you prefer more vegetables than fruit, you can request green capsules instead. She says that each batch of Juice Plus is analyzed for standard food grade bacterial count. There have been 23 research studies on Juice Plus. It's a good way to get the recommended 13 fresh fruits and vegetables daily. I will put information about that in the Resource section too.

In addition to her recipe books, *Hungry for Health* and *Hungrier for Health*, Susan also wrote a book called *Vegetable Juices & Cancer Treatment* that you can purchase at her website: www.beatcancer.org. She says that the research shows that a heavily based plant diet, low in fat with small amounts of protein, is a terrific anti-cancer diet! Susan recommends trying a juice recipe with spinach, carrot, kale and beet. She warns that toxins may be released and tells people to only store your juices for 12 hours in your fridge.

Some people claim that Dr. Max Gerson reversed cancer in terminal clients with 12 glasses of juice daily. This regime reportedly cleanses the liver, neutralizes cancer-causing free radicals, and enhances immune system functioning. It creates an alkaline environment, which helps decrease acidocis, an acidic condition in the body fluids that allows cancer to thrive. I have not fully examined Gerson's research for myself, but it's worth mentioning in the cancer community because juicing can't hurt and it might help for the recommended reasons.

I also read a book called *The Juice Lady's Turbo Diet* (also in the bibliography). The author gives great vegetable juice recipes and explains that vegetable juices have low sugar, offer an abundance of vitamins, minerals, phytonutrients, and enzymes, and is helpful for weight loss. She cites a study by the Baylor College of Medicine in which a large percentage of participants with Metabolic Syndrome lost weight when adding vegetable juice to their diet—specifically, *four times* the weight of those who did not drink the juice. She recommends you drink juice fresh and store it in a covered jar in the refrigerator for up to 24 hours only.

WHEATGRASS

Wheatgrass is supposed to be great for cancer. It contains chlorophyll, which has almost the same molecular structure as hemoglobin, and chlorophyll increases hemoglobin production, getting more oxygen to the cancer. Selenium and laetrile are also in wheatgrass, both are anti-cancer. Chlorophyll and selenium also help build your immune system. Furthermore, wheatgrass is one of the most alkaline foods known to mankind.

Wheatgrass contains at least 13 vitamins, including B12, many minerals and trace elements, including selenium, and all 20 amino acids. It also contains the hormone abscisic acid, the antioxidant enzyme SOD (Superoxide Dismutase) and over 30 other enzymes, the antioxidant enzyme cytochrome oxidase, laetrile, and many other nutrients. SOD converts one of the most dangerous free radicals: Reactive Oxygen Species (ROS), into a hydrogen peroxide molecule (which has an extra oxygen molecule to kill cancer cells) and an oxygen molecule.

Research shows that in a study reported in the journal *Mutation Research*, in comparing the anticancer effect of chlorophyll to beta-carotene, and vitamins A, C and E, Chlorophyll was proven to be a more effective antimutagen. It provides oxygen availability, breaks down poisonous carbon dioxide and releases free oxygen.

Most people take wheatgrass immediately after cutting and juicing. The hormone abscisic acid is 40 times more potent *4 hours* after cutting the wheatgrass than it is at the time of cutting. Perhaps you can cut your wheatgrass and juice it. You can drink most of it immediately and then 4 hours later drink the rest.

My sister discovered a health food store near me (even in Brighton Beach) that sells fresh wheatgrass. Kris Carr recommends buying a grinder for $25 and ordering wheatgrass (which lasts a week) to make it yourself. You can order a hand crank grinder for travel at www.healthyjuicer.com. For wheatgrass delivery you can try www.80wheatgrass.com, www.sproutman.com and www.wheatgrass-central.com. I buy it ground already and haven't tried to juice it.

I normally get off the subway at Union Square in Manhattan on Tuesday and Thursday. One day I went in on a Friday and I saw a farmers market there with a wheatgrass stand. A shot of wheatgrass was $3 and you could also buy the fresh wheatgrass if you want to grind or juice on your own. Once you start looking for it, I think you'll be surprised at the number of places where you can find it.

VITAMIN D

Lab research at Rutgers University was published in *Cancer Prevention Research* (2008) where scientists injected rats with breast cancer and then treated them with Gemini 0097 (an active form of Vitamin D3). Gemini 0097 slowed estrogen-positive cancer growth by 60% and estrogen-negative cancer growth by 50%! Some researchers say that 2000 IU of Vitamin D each day can reduce the risk of breast cancer by 50%. It's good to get Vitamin D from the sun or from your diet. Cod liver oil has 1360 IUs per tablespoon, so you could have this daily. One egg yolk also has 25 IUs of Vitamin D.

OTHER

I was reading psychic Michelle Whitedove's books during my treatment and I liked them so much I decided to get a 30-minute psychic reading with her. She won "America's Psychic Challenge" and reportedly has a 98% accuracy rate. My main intention was to explore the emotional or spiritual significance of my cancer. She told me that I'm a testimony to God's grace and my soul knew that my story with cancer would help many women, and that's why I got cancer. She said my book would help a lot of women and said, "I'd put my chips on you!" She told me that my writing was a vehicle so Spirit could work through me and that I would heal and get back to my feisty self soon, but that I needed to rebuild my immune system first because my body had been through a lot. She made some health recommendations that I wanted to share here because they're good ideas! I'm sure my oncologist would laugh if he knew I was taking health advice from a psychic but I am open to healing from most sources as long as it works for me.

10 HEALTH RECOMMENDATIONS (PER MICHELLE WHITEDOVE)

1. *Don't use deodorant with aluminum.* Buy "Toms" brand instead. Others clog the lymph nodes

2. *Buy organic food—especially chicken and cheese.* Non-organic chicken and cheese are loaded with steroids and antibiotics

3. *Take acidophilus which helps rebuild the immune system if you have yeast proliferation.* Take 3 in morning, 3 at night. Yeast builds up. It's an allergic reaction from inside. She says that if things are heavy on your tummy this can lead to fatigue and Epstein Barr and fibromyalgia

4. *Eat browns instead of whites*—this includes brown bread, brown rice and wheat pasta

5. *Stay away from caffeine*

6. *Eat small meals 4-6 times a day*

7. *Don't eat late at night*

8. *Buy Peptides sachets* that are listed on her website under Links, from Wolfe farms. 1 Peptide sachet bag boosts your immune system for a week. Put it in water for 15 minutes and then drink it. Buy 5 of them and follow this schedule. Use Bag 1 right away. Use Bag 2 the following week. Wait one more week and then use Bag 3. Wait 2 weeks and then take Bag 4. Wait 3 weeks then take Bag 5. Each sachet is $55 each, so 5 are a total of $275

9. *Drink alkaline water, like the Essentia water* I was drinking

10. Go to Manatec website and order *glyco bears* and take 2 a day each

Thanks Michelle! XOXO

Inflammation

Acute inflammation is characterized by the redness, heat, swelling, and pain that is the immune system's normal response to infection or injury. Immune cells congregate at the site so that they can dispose of infectious organisms. But there is also low-grade, chronic inflammation as well, which may underlie a "unified field" explanation of disease.

There is an easy way to test for low-level chronic inflammation, since it can prompt the liver to produce a protein in the blood known as C-reactive protein (CRP). Elevated levels of CRP often accompany or signal an increased risk of heart attack and stroke.

In terms of inflammation-causing foods, I read that for many people this includes red meat, corn, margarine, red and green peppers, citrus fruit, wheat, eggs, sugar, salt and coffee. But, it's best to learn how your body responds to each food.

In Kris Carr's workshop she went over a checklist for inflammation that she uses with clients. It may be helpful for you to consider these questions and to look at which area you first want to address. You can rate each answer from 1-10 (10 being the most):

- What is your energy level?

- What is your stress level?

- How much time do you spend in nature?
- How much movement do you do?
- How much do you drink caffeine—soda, coffee and tea?
- How much do you drink alcohol?
- How much water do you drink?
- How much do you sleep?
- How much dairy do you eat?
- How much sugar do you it?
- How much gluten do you eat?
- How good is your support system?
- How much vacation/ leisure do you have?

How did you do? What areas could you address to decrease your inflammation level? Could you spend more time in nature, decrease stress, lessen caffeine, eliminate sugar, sleep more or which one? Take a moment to journal and make a plan.

Detoxification

After I completed chemotherapy and radiation and had the port removed, I felt really lousy. I knew that my immune system was weakened and I'd also been told that if my cancer spread it would be terminal and they would have to treat me with chemotherapy indefinitely. I knew this was my window of opportunity to fully embrace my health.

Do talk with your doctor about a suitable detoxification program you can follow once your chemotherapy and radiation treatments have finished. You have ingested large doses of toxic chemicals and you want to build up your immune system, increase the effectiveness of your organs, and feed your body good nutrients and fuel to recover. Detoxing improves immune function, reduces free radicals, helps destroy cancer cells, clears congestion, and purifies the blood, according to author Cherie Calbom. Over 200 epidemiological studies regarding fruits and vegetables found that a variety of plant foods reduced the risk of nearly every type of cancer. Raw fruits and vegetables are better than cooked or supplements.

I found that one of the best ways to detox and add vegetables into my diet was juicing, and my ongoing goal is to juice daily, or at least three days a week. A helpful book on detoxing is *The Complete Cancer Cleanse* by Calbom, Calom & Mahaffey, which I've listed in the Bibliography section.

If you are willing to pay out of pocket (somewhere over $10,000 per year) Dr. Nicholas Gonzalez in New York City has a nutritional program with supplementation and detoxification that is reported to be very useful. I would have loved to do this program after treatment to detoxify my body but our insurance did not cover it. Dr. Gonzalez's information is in Appendix B if you are interested.

In *The Complete Cancer Cleanse* the process of detoxification is described as removing toxins from the body, toxins that include heavy metals, antibiotics, hormones, anesthetics, drugs, pesticides, chemicals and solvents that are trapped in the body. The authors explain that their program detoxifies the four primary organs of elimination—the liver, the intestines, the kidneys and lungs, and the four channels of elimination—the gallbladder, lymphatic system, the skin and blood.

I loved the idea of all the meds and chemicals going down the drain after all my body had been through. This was a revival period and I needed the energy of raw foods. Authors stress the importance of getting organic whenever possible and I was able to order from FreshDirect so the food came right to my doorstep. Also, wash your produce in the sink. Fill your sink with water and pour 1/4 cup 3 percent hydrogen peroxide into the water. Then soak your produce for 20 minutes and rinse it with clean water. This kills parasites.

I would order kale, Swiss chard, spinach from FreshDirect and it would all barely fit into our refrigerator and it would go bad if I did not remember to wash, cut and make it. So, I started a new system. When it arrived I would wash and cut it up and store it in large zip lock bags in our freezer. This allowed me to easily grab a handful of kale or Swiss chard in the morning to juice. I could also grab a few cups to cook and eat. It was easily stored and saved prep time in the mornings.

You can also order juice and have it delivered. My husband and I went on a date night and found a juice place nearby called "Fuel." It delivered fresh vegetable juices to your house if you order $10 worth, so this was another option when I was rushing or felt lazy.

Coffee Enemas & Colonics

Colonics and coffee enemas are often suggested by cancer survivors as ways to detoxify as well. I waited until I was done my chemotherapy and radiation to try getting the toxins out. Some cancer survivors do 3 coffee enemas a day. I did not have time or discipline for this. Also, an article I read suggested that one should wait at least 3 weeks after chemotherapy before starting coffee enemas, and you should do them gradually because you are releasing chemo chemicals. Talk to your oncologist about how often is right for you. So far, I just tried a colonic once myself. I was busy and couldn't fathom doing it 3 times a day after finally finishing treatment. The good thing is that enemas are inexpensive and can be done at home in less than half an hour. So speak to your doctor and find out what could work for you.

You can also get professional colonics. To clean out the lower part of the colon, enemas are fine. But enemas don't clean about four feet of the colon, so I went to get a professional colonic for $120 at *Love Your Transformation* in New York. The co-owner Cindy worked with me and she seemed very knowledgeable. The colonic was a bit painful (and was definitely uncomfortable) but she talked me through it and I was able to release quite a bit. I had been drinking diet coke for years so there was a lot of gas and acid. She explained some things about vegetable juicing and said they might offer webinars on vegetable juicing in the future. She told me that colonics make a huge difference in health and that when she started to detoxify her own colon she felt lighter emotionally too. She noticed that there was definitely a connection between the things that we physically hang on to and the emotionally toxic feelings and thoughts that we store. She believes that colonics provide a deeper cleansing on multiple levels than enemas can provide.

I have to say that some other doctors are against colonics. They say that they may disturb electrolyte balance and there have been concerns regarding the sanitation of equipment. So ask your doctor but prepare to hear two sides of the colonic argument, depending on who you speak to. This can be confusing for patients who want to help heal themselves after treatment.

I can't tell you what to do. Maybe there are people who suffered adversely from colonics but I happened to read a few cases from cancer survivors who benefited from them. You will need to decide for yourself. I will put a few NYC resources in the Appendix but you can search your area for practitioners near you if you decide to try it. If you want to try an enema at home, (which I have not yet done) check out www.thewellnesswarrior.com.au. Jessica Ainscough has a YouTube video that walks you through how to do a coffee enema and also sells a guide on her website which explains it. Don't do this at night because it may interfere with your sleep.

Why do all this, you might ask? Well, reportedly coffee enemas eliminate toxins through the liver and increase bile output. This alkalinizes the small intestines and cleans your colon's walls. It enhances digestion and removes toxins in your large intestine. Talk to your doctor about it first to make sure it won't be harmful.

Environmental Toxins & Electromagnetic Fields

Environmental factors are said to cause 90% of cancers. The average household and workplace contain about 62 toxic chemicals used on a daily basis. Our air is polluted, our water has fluoride, aluminum and other chemicals. We have toxins from cleaning supplies, artificial sweeteners, fructose corn syrup, and any of these can cause cellular destruction, which can lead to cancer.

I switched mostly to Seventh Generation cleaners because they aren't toxic. You can also use white vinegar, baking soda, and hydrogen peroxide to clean/disinfect almost everything. It's easy and inexpensive and safe.

I also try to buy organic fruits and veggies to stay away from pesticides. There are also synthetic chemicals in cosmetics cleaners and plastics. We must educate ourselves about this because many say that our environment and those toxins are part of the cause of the rise of cancer rates.

The U.S. Environmental Protection Agency has found a link between electromagnetic fields and cancer. *In Energy Medicine* Donna Eden explains that extended exposure to high-intensity electromagnetic fields has been associated with increased incidence of Alzheimer's disease, depression, suicide, leukemia and cancers of the blood, breast, lung, brain, colon, prostate, lymph and nervous system. She says, "The barrage of artificial electric and magnetic fields can harden cell membranes, alter DNA, and adversely impact hormone production and neurological processes (leading to) more rapid aging, elevated blood glucose levels, elevated lipid levels high blood pressure, increased neuron-regulatory disturbances and it compromises the central nervous, cardiovascular and immune systems."

In *The Promise of Energy Psychology* Donna Eden's husband David Feinstein says that any substance your immune system does not recognize may disrupt your energy system. He says that we are exposed to at least 15,000 artificial chemicals in our food alone. We also breathe fumes from our cars, smoke stacks, and insulation in our homes. Donna cites research that telephone linemen experience elevated electromagnetic fields and have as much as a six-fold incidence of certain types of cancer!

Cellphones and computers can have safe screens. You can use glass plates and mugs instead of ceramic ones because some ceramics contain lead. You can get cosmetics and shampoos that are natural in health food stores and research the ingredients. You can use Seventh Generation cleaners in your home that aren't harmful.

David Schmidt of "Life Wave" created a device called a nanotechnology patch of glutathione that you can wear daily to detox your body of cancer-causing free radicals. Suzanne Somers uses it and recommends it in her book Knockout. See the Reference section for website information about this device.

You can check out www.emfpollution.com to learn more about this subsection.

Recreation

I put recreation and the next few subcategories under this Body section because much of the physical things we do for fun seem to fit here and raise our frequency.

Our body needs to recharge and have fun: creating a great environment and socializing can engage our parasympathetic nervous system. I've included a few suggestions below that may help—and are fun too!

Feng Shui

For it is only framed in space that beauty blossoms.

Anne Morrow Lindberg

Have you ever noticed that when you have a relaxing environment, your body relaxes too? So does your Spirit. Perhaps you've noticed that when your space is uncluttered, your mind is also clear? Feng shui masters help the energy in your environment to flow properly. Some say this corresponds to the energy flow in your body.

Psychoanalyst Carl Jung said that when you dream of going into different rooms in a house, it's really a dream about going into different parts of yourself. Many healers say that our physical "stuff" accumulates in our energy body as an extension of what we have to manage and carry, and if we don't address it, it can move into our physical body as disease. Thus, going through and getting rid of stuff that you don't need can be uplifting, freeing, and may possibly be good for your physical health too.

I eventually got into the swing of things with clearing and organizing our apartment during my cancer treatments. We had been struggling to work, clean, and do the laundry each week, and my mom found a wonderful young woman to clean for $15 an hour on a weekend. She loved to organize and picked up some storage bins to help me get started. We started with one closet and then I was inspired to continue when she wasn't there. I ended up speaking to a friend on the phone while I reorganized my bookshelves and the linen closet.

Creating order during a time of such chaos felt good. Creating space physically also allows energies to flow, so new things can come into your life. It also gives you the added benefit of gifting things you no longer use to people who will value them. Plus, having a clear, peaceful space is so important in terms of refueling and honoring yourself. Your home is your nest and your place to regenerate.

So, I would suggest getting a fun helper and starting to think about how you can make your environment more conscious and comfortable. If this feels like pressure or something "you have to do" during this challenging time, then skip it. You are tired during treatment and don't need more pressure. But if you can do it in increments or you'd enjoy it, this can be a great way to rebalance your energy, inside and outside.

Vacation

I must remember to see
with island eyes.

Anne Morrow Lindberg

Especially in this day and age, our bodies need rest and time to refuel. Our minds need a break and our adult Spirits need play time too. This is what a vacation is for!

Most people probably won't take a big vacation during treatment because during chemotherapy they are too scared something will happen to their health. They fear that they won't be near the hospital and during radiation they need to be at the hospital on a daily basis. However, it can be a great idea to take a mini-break and go to a bed and breakfast, or a spa during the weekend.

Also, some people dream of traveling when they get sick with cancer. They are more likely to want to see the world, in case their time is limited. It can be inspiring to read up on places and plan some trip itineraries for when you are finished treatment and feeling up to traveling again. This planning and dreaming can be inspiring.

And, after you are done with treatment, I definitely recommend a vacation as a reward! As I write, this, I will be finishing treatment in October, and my husband and I plan to go away for a short trip and then a five-day getaway in February for our 6th wedding anniversary. I can't wait! It's fun to have a positive reward at the end of your journey.

Regular Play Time

Life must be lived as play.

PLATO

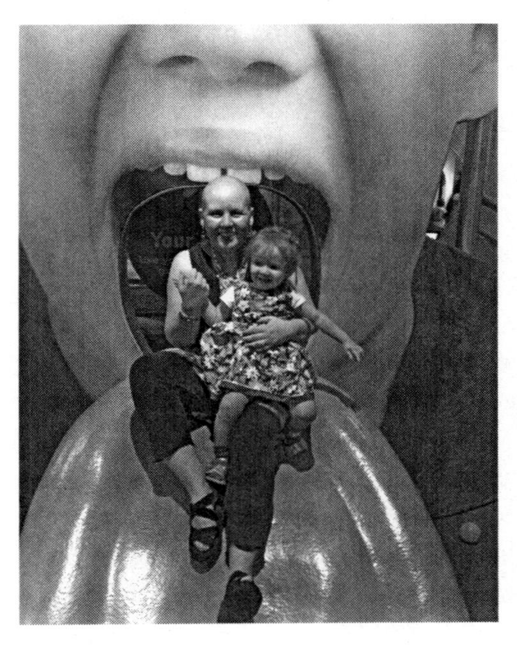

HERE IS A PICTURE OF ME WITH MY DAUGHTER, SERA, AT THE CHILDREN'S MUSEUM IN MANHATTAN. WE ARE SLIDING DOWN A TONGUE TOGETHER! ANYTHING YOU CAN DO TO PLAY AND LAUGH DURING YOUR CANCER TREATMENT IS GOOD.

My son Noble had his 4th birthday party at "Bounce U" in Brooklyn and my husband and I jumped with the kids in the bouncy houses, and slid down those giant slides. We had a ball. My wig almost fell off but I felt great. It occurred to me that hospitals should unite to hold a Bounce U event for patients going through cancer treatment, since laughter is so therapeutic.

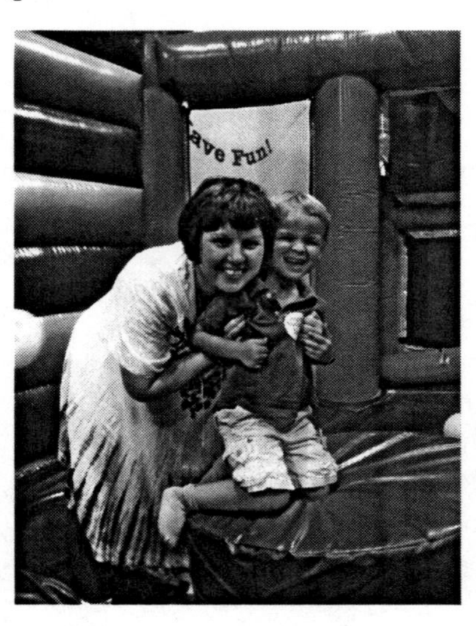

THIS IS MY SON NOBLE AND I AT HIS BOUNCE U PARTY.

Kids are the best people to remind you of how to play, let go, be present and have fun. If you don't have a child, maybe you can borrow one!

If you are single, you can try singing, dancing, taking belly dancing, going to comedy shows or seeing friends. Find out what kinds of play or creativity that you love and do it at least twice a week.

Spiritually speaking, play is God. In *The Path to Love* Deepak Chopra writes, "Survival is too pressing an issue for us to feel that our life is pure play. But in spirit you only play. Your purpose is not to survive but to express every grain of passion that love arouses in you." I love that!

Date Night

Romance is everything.

Gertrude Stein

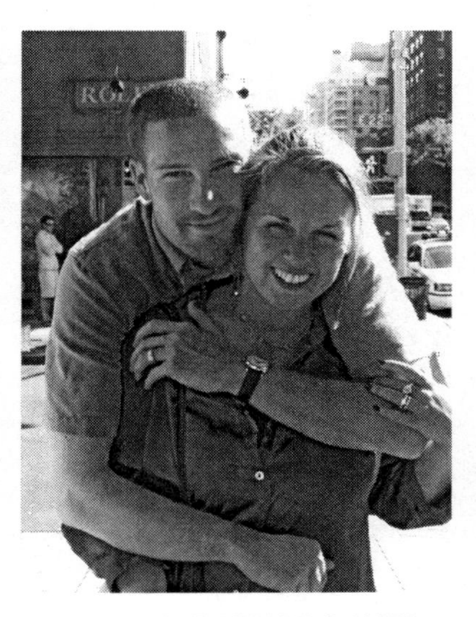

DATE NIGHT BEFORE CANCER

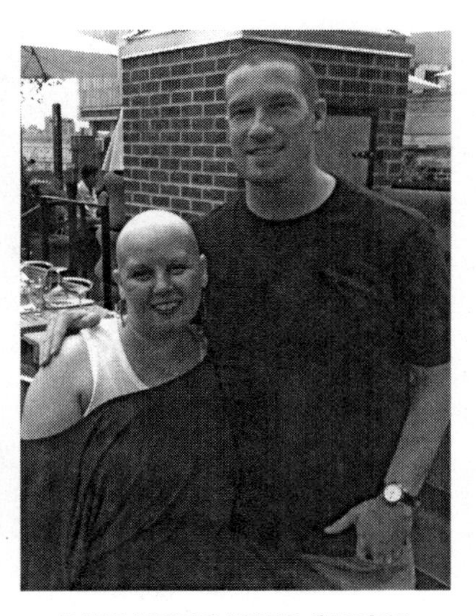

DATE NIGHT AFTER CANCER

Sometimes when people have cancer they isolate and become homebodies because they are bald, tired, and symptomatic. Romance goes out the widow and partners drift apart. Don't let this happen!

You can still feel loveable and beautiful, and hopefully your partner will remind you of that.

I put this under the Body section because Date night can involve dancing, eating, and physical affection.

I suggest a weekly or at least bi-weekly date night. I would go out bald sometimes if my wig was too hot. It felt great to leave responsibilities behind and just spend some time with my husband. Sometimes he'd order a glass of wine and I'd have iced tea with Stevia, but it was still fun. Maybe you'll even receive some pretty flowers, like I did.

See below:

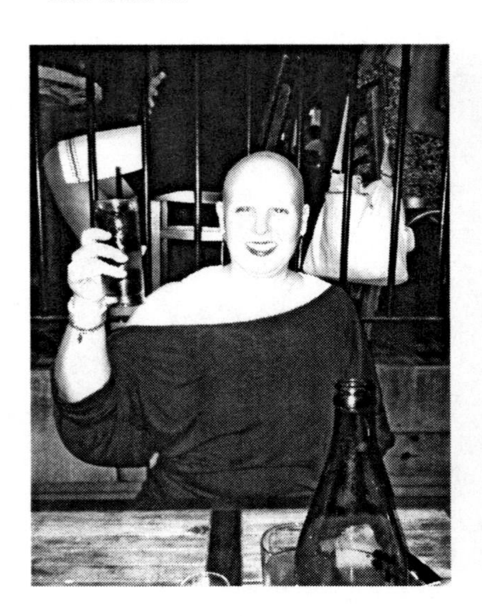

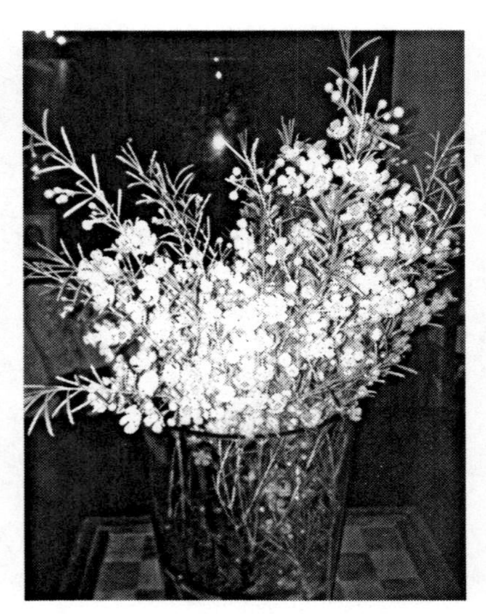

And if you're single you can still buy yourself flowers and go dancing with a friend.

I imagine it would be hard to date and try to meet someone during your treatment year but I have heard stories where it's happened. In Kris Carr's *Crazy Sexy Cancer Tips* she documents how she met and started dating the man who is now her husband, after she was diagnosed with cancer. They are now married and are considering trying to have a child. There are even dating sites for people with cancer. If you are interested in dating other cancer survivors or people with illness, check out www.cisforcupid.com, www.cancermatch.com, www.prescription4love.com or www.cancerpatientmingle.com.

As a dating coach, I also think you could sign up for a general site such as www.eharmony.com, www.match.com or www.okcupid.com and let people know what you are going through, either in your profile or after a few dates. The point is that you can choose to be open to attracting love and support at any time. Remember that you are beautiful (even without hair) and you will not be going through this forever. Hopefully life, love, and romance will return to normal soon, but sometimes it comes to us in unexpected times and ways too.

Celebrate and Take a Vacation!

The more you praise and celebrate your life,
the more there is in life to celebrate.

Oprah Winfrey

Celebration is great for your body and immune system. Celebrating life brings in laughter and good endorphins, reminding you of how glad you are to be here.

When I finished my 8 chemotherapies and 33 radiation treatments my husband planned a road trip over a long weekend to celebrate. We drove 7 hours to Lilydale, NY to see the psychic and then drove to Niagara Falls. We had a great time!

Here are some websites that offer free vacations to cancer survivors. I did not use them but they might be good resources for you:

Karen Wellington Foundation for LIVING with Breast Cancer (www.karenwellingtonfoundation.org) an organization in honor of Karen Wellington that gives vacations to cancer survivors.

Send Me On Vacation (www.sendmeonvacation.org) an organization that picks some cancer survivors and awards them up to $1500 for a vacation.

Stowe Weekend of Hope (www.stowehope.org) a weekend of free hotels and workshops in Vermont for cancer survivors. This year it's in May 2013 and you can register in February.

Maybe if you can't get away overnight you can just plan an evening out with friend!

The day I finished my last radiation treatment my husband brought home chocolate cupcakes with sprinkles (although this may seem ironic given my new healthy eating path) and my family sang, "Happy Cancer-Free Day to you" to me. I made a wish for radiant health and happiness and blew out the candle. See below:

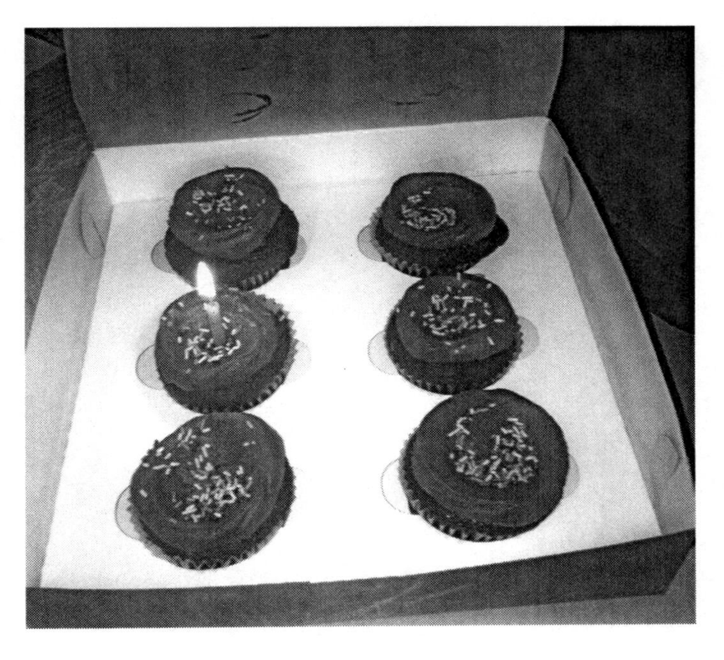

OUR "HAPPY CANCER-FREE DAY TO YOU!" PARTY

What will *you* do when you're all done?

SECTION II

Mind

This is your world. Shape it or someone else will.

Gary Lew

The mental body is supposedly the one I was in too much! I spent a lot of time in my mind, analyzing things and solving problems. I'd sit in a chair all day with my patients or write at my computer. My mind was nearly all that existed. My spiritual mentor Christopher says there is an irony: the more intelligent your mind is, the easier it is to be trapped there.

My job was to merge my mind with my heart and Spirit, and in this section we will discuss some ways our thoughts and mental body might affect the manifestation of illness and how we can use our thoughts to heal instead.

Studies show how much our mind and thoughts do influence our body. Deepak Chopra discusses a study done on Tibetan monks in his book, *Reinventing Your Body, Resurrecting the Soul.* This study was done in cooperation with the Dalai Lama and it allowed brain researchers to study advanced Buddhist monks who had been meditating between 15–40 years. In the laboratory these monks were hooked up to functional MRIs and asked to meditate on compassion. They generated the most intense gamma waves ever seen in a normal brain. Gamma waves are associated with keeping the brain functioning as a whole and with higher order thinking. The most intense area of activity was in their left prefrontal cortex, which is the area associated with happiness and positive thoughts. This demonstrated that mental activity alone could alter the brain.

Chopra gives another example of the connection between mind and body when he describes the Tibetan meditation called *tumo*, which protects the body from the elements. These monks can sit in caves overnight at subzero temperatures in a silk robe and emerge unaffected. The monks raised their internal temperatures by 8 degrees Fahrenheit, a heat that affects the hypothalamus. Other yogis train themselves in meditation to need only minimal food, and have been buried in coffins for days, surviving on very little air by lowering their breathing rates and basal metabolism.

Most of us have not developed this level of awareness and control! But reading these studies on what is possible through meditation I thought how much it could benefit our society to teach meditation in schools, so that children could learn how to monitor their thoughts and impulses, and understand the relationship between thoughts, feelings, and their bodies. This could end up being an 11-year training, from 1st grade through high school. What results might be possible!

Studies originating at the School of Engineering at Princeton University suggest thoughts affect subtle energies. Other studies confirm that some individuals can consistently provide an accurate medical diagnosis from a distance. For example, on a sample of 50 patients of Dr. Norman Shealy's, Carolyn Myss's clairvoyant diagnosis (from a distance) matched his in 93% of the diseases identified.

In *Energy Medicine* Donna Eden explains there is growing evidence that certain subtle energies are Quantum Fields, "non-local" in their effects, so distance doesn't affect them. Thus, our thoughts have much more power than we ever realized. As we increase our awareness of our thoughts, we may be better able to affect how our bodies respond, as well as diagnose ourselves.

One of the best things I did toward "mental healing" was to get an iPhone and download healing apps and CDs onto my cell phone. This way, when I was running around or in transit, I could use that time to learn or practice a guided meditation. I would walk the beach and listen to a lecture by Marianne Williamson, or do the Sedona Method during a break. The mental body is a key aspect of how we can learn, grow, and acquire wisdom and divine guidance.

In *Knockout*, Dr. Stephen Sinatra says that the most important element for cancer survivors is the belief that they can get well. He tries to instill that belief in patients and encourages other doctors to be positive and hopeful as well. Bruce Lipton (Biology of Belief) says that if your intention and belief are strong enough you can even change your DNA.

I was fortunate that I believed (most of the time) I was going to be fine and fully recover from the cancer, so I did not drain too much energy dealing with fear. But sometimes you can be too much in your mind, to the exclusion of your heart and soul, and this creates energetic imbalance. I was very entrenched in my mind in the past few years. My mind was king, but Christopher suggested that instead I think of my Soul as king, my heart as queen, and my mind as a knight that served the royal couple. Often my mind was the same as my ego. It wanted order, control, and linear thinking. This cancer path showed me that this is a very limited way to view the world, and that imposing arbitrary limitations on life can make it harder to deal with events and circumstances that seem to be out of our control—such as cancer!

In this Mind section, I will explore some tools that serve us and some negative thinking styles that sabotage us on life's journey.

Your thoughts are key in determining your emotions and actions so work hard on making them constructive but remember to keep your sense of humor. As Dr. Seuss reminds us, we can control our thoughts playfully. He says, "Think left and think right and think low and think high. Oh, the thinks you can think up if only you try!"

The Inner Critic/Gremlin

The world is the mirror image of your mind.

Byron Katie

We don't realize how often we criticize ourselves. Chris says this is worse than radiation. There's compelling evidence that negative thoughts may poorly affect our cells.

Joyce Hawkes, a biophysicist, cellular healer and author of *Cell Level Healing*, says that cell sap, called cytoplasm, is 90% water—and our thoughts can affect this cell water and our critical life functions. Masuru Emoto, a Doctor of Alternative Healing has done extensive work on the effects of thoughts on water, and believes that negative thinking negatively affects the crystalline structure of water.

We have 60,000 thoughts a day and probably 90% of them (for the average person) are negative. Christopher says that when the mind gives you critical thoughts and wants to be "King of the Hill" you can just say, "Mind, thank you for sharing." You need to practice a lot and be consistent. He makes the analogy that feeding your trash thoughts by trying to "understand them" is worse than eating junk food! The remedy is to simply notice when a negative thought shows up, and to replace it with a thought that returns you to trusting love and light.

Sometimes your inner critic is worried about what other people think about you. In *A Thousand Names for Joy*, Byron Katie says, "When you open your arms to criticism, you are your own direct path to freedom, because you can't change us or what we think about you. You are your only way to stand with a friend as a friend, even when she perceives you as an enemy. And until you can be intimate with us however badly we think of you, your Work isn't done." When you love yourself unconditionally no matter what others think of you, then you have done your work.

Begin to notice when you are judging yourself or others, or are paying attention to others judging you. Hale Dwoskin, the creator of the "Sedona Method" says, "If you are "shoulding"on yourself or someone else, release instead. You can always choose to let whatever it is and refocus on love and peace."

Our Gremlin is critical and judgmental because its main job is to keep us safe. It is the inner critic that doesn't like growth or change. If we want to evolve we need to dialogue with our Gremlin so we can let love in and allow our Spirit to remain in charge.

Here's an example of an exercise I often give my clients to deal with their Gremlin. Let's take a scenario where someone wants to sing at a concert but her Gremlin is telling her that no one will like her performance or voice. She is journaling a dialogue here between her Gremlin (G) and her Higher Self (HS):

GREMLIN EXERCISE

G: Susan, just stay home. Your life is fine. Why would you want to sing and make a fool of yourself?

HS: I love singing and expressing myself.

G: Are you crazy? Just sing in the shower? Why risk it? You're not even getting paid!

HS: I don't want to hide or live my life in fear. I want to share my gifts and I don't need to be perfect to be loveable. I will be okay!

You can carry around your journal and do this kind of dialogue to externalize that critical internal voice and challenge it. It may seem silly but it's also very powerful and it allows your Higher Self to stay in charge and reveals inner thoughts that we hadn't previously known or paid attention to.

Your Wounded Child

The only reason that you want to understand your problems is because you're planning to have them again.

Hale Dwoskin

Even if you had a great childhood, most of us have within us a wounded child who acts out or remains frustrated in some way. As Carolyn Myss says, "Your biography becomes your biology." Many of us have a wounded inner child that has been ignored, and that unexplored emotion can wreak havoc with our body.

In her book, *Emergence*, Barbara Marx Hubbard describes how at 70 years old her inner mother healed her wounded child. She was able to do this by spending time in unconditional love and stillness, listening to the voice of her wounded child and giving it wisdom and compassion. She says, "Whenever a local self acts up, feels stress, hurt, anger, anxiety or fear, we can learn to radiate the inner presence upon that wounded self." By doing this for two hours a day, within a year she experienced a profound shift from ego to essence, from anxiety to bliss.

In *True Love* Thich Nhat Hanh says, "When the mother hears her baby crying, she puts down whatever she has in her hands, she goes into its room and takes the baby in her arms . . . it loses energy every time it is embraced by the energy of mindfulness, which is really a mother."

By paying attention to the wounded child, making her safe and comforting her, the child can quiet down.

I spoke to Chris about my wounded child. He intuited a 4-year-old girl that he called "the rebel." She felt entitled not to follow the rules, doesn't want to sleep, exercise, or eat right. She just says, "Because I'm right!" and she also says, "You can't make me!" Chris asked me, "Is that the game you want to play every day? She is forming an ingrained habit. She keeps you unconscious. She thinks God will punish her when she is bad and in a way she wants God to prove that he can heal her cancer without her doing *anything*, but God helps those who help themselves. In a way, she loved the cancer treatment because she could still do what she wanted due to the power of science, chemotherapy, and radiation. Your job is to love her and be there for her in union so she doesn't have to rebel anymore. Don't cast her away because she's being annoying. She wants a strong Mother who won't allow her to do what's bad for her. Be willing to be with her so her fear goes away and you are then free to make better choices. We are here to perfect ourselves and change negative habits."

This seemed like good advice. I can't say I'm going to be fanatically good about eating healthfully but I will try to skew towards doing what is loving for myself and continue to notice when I choose the "shadow" path, so I can then have the choice to move back towards my Source.

The Wounded Child often acts out when you are scared, so she may need extra attention on a chemotherapy or radiation day or on a day that she is particularly sad or lonely. When you are practicing soothing your Wounded Child you might try some tapping as well: Feinstein suggests that tapping acupoints while saying soothing words during the heat of an incident can quickly calm a person.

RESTRUCTURING

I did a healing session with Tom Cratsley, who used a method that he calls *Restructuring.* Tom describes Restructuring as looking at unconscious resistance patterns and noticing how they are held and how they limit us. Through regression and a series of relieving statements about choices and old emotions, you change how you relate to the trauma or memory. I told him that I was exploring any unconscious reasons for getting breast cancer right now. He intuited that there was some kind of self-nurturing component and suggested that we start the process. We did this session by phone.

He asked me to notice where in my body there was tension and to be willing to go deeper into it. I counted back from 5 to 0 and went deeper into any physical and emotional discomfort until I arrived at what I sensed was the first time I may have created this conflict.

As I did this I remembered a few situations from childhood and a series of choices, emotions, and limiting beliefs that surfaced. I saw myself in a series of scenes with my sister and my mother fighting, and I was trying to be the peacemaker. One belief or choice I made then was, *If I'm not on top of things, things will go crazy without me.* I told that little girl that now she can be okay around other people's craziness without having to intervene. She could let adults handle their own upset and problems. She had also decided, *"When other people have problems, there's no room for me to be or have what I want."* I now assured her that she could have relationships where there was room for her desires and who she was, so she could be fully expressed and appreciated. She had also told herself, *"I can only get along with others by caring for their needs without regard for my own."* I released all that was said and done to support that conclusion as well.

There was also a scene at 16 years old where I felt like I had failed at my self-imposed job as "Peacemaker" because my parents divorced after 22 years of marriage. I had to forgive myself for not doing the job I expected to do and release any judgment that it was my job in the first place or that I had failed.

The little 4-year-old girl and the 16-year-old was angry at her parents, for being sad and unhealed in their own ways and for letting her/me take on those responsibilities or encouraging me in that role. My parents used to call me "Sunshine" because I was the one who tried to cheer everyone up. I forgave them for their insensitivities. The little girl also forgave my sister for being the "problem child" because she felt that she never got as much attention because of this.

Ultimately, this little girl felt like there was no room for her to be the person she wanted to be, or to do the things she wanted to do while involved with others. I gave my Wounded Child my blessing to have intimate relationships now that were co-nurturing and collaborative.

When we finished an hour had passed, but it seemed much quicker because I was in an altered state of consciousness. If you'd like to try a Restructuring session, I will put Tom Cratsley's information in the Resource section for you.

In real time, this session reminded me that I needed to make time to nurture myself and not feel that the needs of all my relationships superseded my relationship with myself. I needed to remember to make space for my desires and wishes while the craziness continued in the lives of my loved ones, and to remind myself that there would be love and time enough for self and other in this new balance. I also needed to remember to assert my needs in my relationships. Then my little girl would continue to be heard and healed if I honored her wisdom.

The Chorus of Selves

Our thinking is robbing our experience of a lot of aliveness.

Hale Dwoskin

When I had to spend four hours of daily commuting into the city for radiation treatments, Christopher Dilts recommended that I spend time listening to my inner wisdom about this ordeal, for the next 6 weeks. He suggested that I ask my Higher Self, my Divine Child, My Wounded Child, and My Adult Self for answers so I could learn to differentiate those voices. I decided to try this assignment.

First let me explain these parts:

The *Adult me* is the woman I am now with my ego and personality. Ultimately she's integrated with these other parts for self-actualization but sometimes people never get to that point, and the healing work with the inner child is meant to facilitate this integration.

The *Divine Child* is like a lifetime flower who knows that she is loved and is never in doubt. She's only interested in giving and receiving love and is anchored in sweetness and is in the moment.

The *Wounded Child* is an expression of an inability to trust God. It's our shadow side that feels wounded, alienated and forgotten. It exhibits behaviors of fear, anger, neediness, bitterness, blame, guilt, shame and criticism. When we can understand and integrate our wounded child, she becomes healed.

The *Higher Self* is an eternal part of us that rests in our soul and holds wisdom about our mission and gifts.

One day I was tired and annoyed because all the contacts in my phone had disappeared. I was late to radiation treatment and had not slept. I decided it was a good moment to practice distinguishing these voices and to give each of them a chance to advise me.

I asked my *Divine Self* why I was going through this treatment experience and I heard, "There is a greater purpose and wisdom here than you can see. Just wait. Be patient."

Next I asked my *Divine Child*, who said, "Be in the moment and play with your circumstances. Have fun experiencing something new and find joy in everything you do!"

My *Wounded Child* piped up and said, "This sucks getting up at 5:30 am every day, getting no help and stressing to get to the hospital on time and going through 33 treatments alone!"

The *Adult me* said, "Well, at least you took a car service today and got to stop and grab a bite to eat first. There's a lot of good here too, and today you might even have a chance to nap later!"

We all have these different voices and you can see how many levels of consciousness can operate at once.

One way to choose your vibration and information wisely is to become conscious about which voice is speaking, and when. Then you will be able to choose which information to listen to and which energy is in charge. Otherwise your Wounded Child will automatically take over.

Take some time to identify your own inner voices and notice which one usually is loudest and which is wisest and most helpful.

In order to work on merging these 4 parts of ourselves it helps to invoke the Divine Angelic Matrix first (to be covered in the Angel section later) because support is needed for the Wounded child and for all four parts to be present and merge.

I can imagine many situations where this exercise would be helpful on your path. Whether the focus is your fear of death, your symptoms, your anger at cancer, your fear of being bald, your desire to quit treatment, etcetera, if your Wounded Child becomes too loud, stop and do a dialogue with her, your Divine Child, and your adult self, and discover where it takes you.

Einstein said that you can't solve a problem with the same mind that created it. So, notice when your Wounded self is in charge and help her to raise her vibration and cross over from fear into love. Then journal about your experience and how this helped you.

Anxiety/Stress

Influencing your mind or changing your mental state
can also affect the physiological state of your body.

Dalai Lama

The impact of stress on illness and cancer is another area upon which your healing team may not agree, leaving you to decide for yourself.

When I was first diagnosed, I asked my oncologist at Sloan if stress could trigger the existing cancer cells we have. She replied, "If stress caused cancer then everyone in NYC would have cancer!" It's an amusing line, but there is overwhelming evidence that stress does play a role in lowering the immune system, causing insulin and cortisol levels to rise, increasing inflammation, and causing us to enter into a fight or flight state. My breast surgeon also said that stress did not play a role in getting cancer.

In contrast, many other health professionals feel stress *does* play a big role. By all accounts, it seems to be a healthy thing to address your stress levels anyway, so I felt that it could not hurt and might tremendously help! Shortly I'll provide some stress-busting exercises that I used and that might work for you as well.

In my own life I experienced stress before my diagnosis. I was working a lot, having a few health issues, and my new daughter had a genetic disorder. It was a rare disorder and most doctors had not worked with it before. We attended a conference in Chicago on her disorder and I couldn't help but cry much of the time. Before giving birth to my daughter I had experienced a miscarriage, and a high risk pregnancy with both her and my son, so I'm pretty sure I had some high levels of stress going on.

I asked my social worker at Sloan Kettering what she thought about the role stress could play with cancer, thinking she had seen many cancer patients and would have a well-rounded perspective. She told me that cancer cells couldn't care less if you were a positive or negative person. She said if I try too hard to be positive I will burn out because cancer stinks, so I may as well be realistic and just let myself be sad. She said that stress doesn't affect cancer and thinking that only results in women blaming themselves.

She handed me an article from the New York Times entitled, "Is There a Link Between Stress and Cancer?" published on November 29, 2005 and written by Gina Kolata. The article said that researchers have explored whether stress might suppress immune system cells needed to kill cancer cells. A tenuous connection between stress, the immune system, and cancer emerged because it appears that cancer cells make proteins that actually tell the immune system to leave them alone or to help them grow!

The article covered a lot of ground about there being no clear connection between stress and cancer though.

According to research cited in this article, other studies say there is no clear connection between stress and cancer. Polly Newcomb, the head of cancer prevention programs at Fred Hutchinson Cancer Center Research Center in Seattle used trained interviewers to ask women with cancer and healthy women as controls about their medical history, environments and medications. She asked 1000 women about stressful life events and found no association between stressful life events in the previous 5 years and the diagnosis of breast cancer.

Large studies of cancer and stress were also done in Denmark where they looked at the incidence of cancer in 11,380 parents of children with cancer, but the parents themselves had no greater incidence of cancer than the general population. This pointed to the fact that these parents' stress concerning their children made them no more likely to contract cancer themselves.

According to Dr. Drew Pardoll, the director of cancer immunology program at John Hopkins Kimmel Comprehensive Cancer Center, the white blood cells of the immune system always bump into cancer cells and try to destroy them. But stress can weaken the immune system and hinder this surveillance. However, Dr. Fred Appelbaum, Director of the clinical research division at the Fred Hutchinson Center found when they studied mice that were genetically engineered with *no* immune system, the common types of cancer were not increased.

So, does stress affect cancer or not? Counselors and doctors probably do not want patients to blame themselves and to think that their stress caused their own cancer. It's true that many anxious people never get cancer, but to my mind it can't hurt to give your immune system a great boost by activating your sympathetic nervous system, reducing your stress, and increasing peace of mind and body.

Other studies and healers suggest there *is* a correlation between stress and cancer:

Susan Silberstein feels that there is a link between mental/emotional states and susceptibility to a breast cancer diagnosis: stress affects our nervous system, alters immunological response, and affects our hormones. Susan cites a Study at Seattle Cancer Research Center, which showed cancerous tumors that developed in 60% of mice in stressful surroundings compared with 7% protected from environmental stress. This was especially true when there was prolonged emotional stress. Susan says that when she has interviewed over 10,000 breast cancer patients, 95% without hesitation said that their disease came from stress.

Hans Selye, a pioneer in stress research felt that all of us have a limited quantity of energy available for the body to adapt to both physical and mental trauma. He felt that if too much energy was used for mental trauma, we'd lower our immune system and couldn't handle our physical needs.

In the early 1960s, psychiatrists Holmes and Rahe noticed a high percentage of cancer patients had experienced pretty severe psychological trauma between 6-18 months before diagnosis. They felt that if there was a connection between these two events, and trauma was necessary to weaken the immune system and permit illness, they might be able to predict who would become ill. They created the Holmes-Rahe Social Readjustment Scale and did a year-long study. Forty-nine percent of the people who had experienced traumatic events the preceding year (who had a cumulative score of over 300 in terms of trauma) suffered a serious illness after. Only 9% of those who scored 200 and below became ill in the same period.

Joyce Hawkes, author of *Cell-Level Healing* says that stress induces depression of the immune system and reduces nerve regeneration, which can block the body's healing.

Stress is often induced by great changes and many people experience change before a cancer diagnosis. In one study, monkeys were put into stressful circumstances to see what happened to them physiologically. Five caged monkeys who previously hadn't seen each other were put in a cage together. Monkeys normally choose a commander monkey and they determine who the leader will be by fighting. Every two months, the researchers took out two monkeys so they had to fight again to see who would be the commander monkey. This rotation of monkeys happened for a year. There was also a control group of monkeys with no fighting or changes in their commander. The group of monkeys *with* the changes developed blocked arteries. The boss monkey in the change group had the worst heart disease of all the monkeys but the boss monkey in the non-change group had the least. This can lead you to believe that change and stress often does have physical consequences.

Researchers at Ohio State University looked at medical students studying for major exams and therefore were under stress. The students showed large drops in their lymphatic t-cell and b-cell levels, and had many colds and flus.

Donna Eden says, "Stress has an immediate impact on every system in your body . . . The daily stresses of life trigger the primitive brain centers into an emergency response condition, up to 80 percent of the blood leaves our forebrain to support the fight-or-flight response, stress chemicals pour into our bloodstream, primitive stress-response emotions sweep over us." Eden recommends that we learn how to hold specific spots on our head called neurovascular holding points for 1-5 minutes in order to reset our nervous system when we are stressed. She describes this further in her book on pages 102-103.

So, which is it? Many people thrive on clear rules and prescriptions for life and behavior. I personally prefer order and control but cancer is a teacher in so many ways. It teaches us to sit with paradox and to look at both sides of an equation and decide for ourselves. Life isn't black and white. We are each different in how we experience and cope with stress—especially the stress of cancer.

Some tools to help deal with stress include meditation, self-monitoring, stimulus control, behavioral self-regulation, and cognitive therapy. Drawing from the description of these tools by Daniel Brown in *Healing Emotions*, here are some approaches you can try:

Self-monitoring: keep a daily diary of your symptoms and rate them 0-5 for pain. Note what you're doing, thinking, and feeling at those times and see if there are any patterns.

Stimulus Control: habits become associated with neutral events through learning. For example, you start thinking about pain before radiation therapy and then get a headache.

Behavioral Self-regulation: you can self-monitor your habits and begin to cut them down. You can work out a schedule and goals and work towards this. For example, if you drink 5 diet cokes a day and know they are bad for your cancer, you can work out a schedule where each month you eliminate one soda a week.

Cognitive Therapy: by journaling your thoughts you can challenge them and develop an antidote to them.

Another easy tool that I use with my clients, I call, "The Facts or the Story." I ask them to differentiate the facts from the story they make up about it. So, for example, a client tells me that a new boyfriend said that he would call her after they'd been dating a few months, but he did not. The fact is that *he did not call.* The story my client might make up about this fact is that he is having an affair, or that he is leaving the relationship. If we rate the level of distress just from the fact, "he did not call her," the client reports a 5 out of 10. If we add her story, "He is permanently breaking up with me," the stress level becomes a 10 out of 10. Plus, the story is not reality because the lack of calling could have been something benign like him falling asleep or being stuck at a work event.

Try this simple exercise the next time you exacerbate your stress by creating a negative story around an event related to your cancer. Deconstruct it and make sure that you are not catastrophizing and getting ahead of yourself! This small exercise is very helpful.

SOME STRESS RESOURCES

In terms of addressing your stress, there is a DVD called *A Meditation to Help You Fight Cancer* by Belleruth Naparstek that you can order on Amazon. It provides healing imagery and guided meditation to mobilize immune response, shrink tumors, and expand love and gratitude.

I am working on a CD called *Cancer Path Meditations*. You can learn more about this on my website www.thecancerpath.com. It has helpful affirmations and meditations to help you maintain a positive frame of mind throughout your treatment.

As you progress in your spiritual development and gain faith in Spirit and your Higher self, your anxiety will diminish because as you feel loved and safe almost all the time. Barbara Marx Hubbard describes this transformation in her book *Emergence*. Meditating for three hours every day eventually led to her integrating the "essence" state of consciousness into her daily life. She discusses how her anxiety diminished saying, "My nervous system stopped being irritated by compulsive thoughts. The constant feeling of being rushed slowly but surely faded. If I awoke with the old twang of anxiety, I recalled my experience of the beloved and the nervousness seemed to disappear... The moment you feel a pang of ego expressing through anxiety, irritation anger-stop. Breathe. Return to essence . . . For spiritual athletes, this is a vital ongoing practice." I like the idea that the challenge of cancer is encouraging us to become spiritual athletes.

For me, anxiety often had to do with racing thoughts, getting ahead of myself, or rushing. My Gremlin often told me there was no time to get anything done. Meditating helped me slow down, breathe and get present. Barbara Marx Hubbard says, "Focus on the beloved and allow that presence to lift you up. We need to slow down to accomplish our rendezvous with destiny." I love the paradox of slowing down in order to get where we most want to go. It's an epiphany for most New Yorkers!

When I remember to meditate I start my day with a blank mental state, with inspiring energy, with more centeredness and with a knowing that I have already done something good for myself. I find that I am more present, less irritable, more patient and better able to hear messages from my Higher self.

Monkey-Mind Attachments

*I have heard there are troubles of more than one kind.
Some come from ahead and some come from behind. But I've
bought a big bat. I'm all ready you see. Now my troubles
are going to have troubles with me!*

Dr. Seuss

I had a session with Christopher Dilts and he told me a story about monkeys. He said sometimes there is something a monkey wants and it's in a jar. So the monkey jams his hand into the jar to grab it. As a result, the monkey cannot get his hand out of the jar and he won't let go. The monkey 's ego won't resist, so its hand remains stuck. More than 2000 years ago Buddha said that wanting was the source of suffering. How will you acknowledge this wanting in your life?

Christopher and I joked about making a Monkey Jar Inventory. I asked myself: What is my Monkey-Mind attached to that isn't serving me? It would probably still be a long list even though I've made a lot of changes.

My monkey-mind ego was attached to diet coke, to sugar and carbs to some extent, to arguing with Ian about date night, to overworking, being a successful author, and making this world a better place.

Once I became aware—conscious—of this, I could decide what to let go of. Was the cookie the booby prize?

Before you read on, take a moment and make a list of your own Monkey Jar inventory. Where in your life do you keep reaching for things that get you stuck and don't serve you? How might you stop or shift this practice? Hale Dwoskin, founder of the Sedona Method says that you can want something without craving results. This means you want something but you're not emotionally attached to whether you get it or not. This is a good mindset to aim for. Stop throughout your day and notice what results you are still overly attached to and why. In *The Path to Love* Deepak Chopra says, "Attachment is that condition in which your needs overshadow your spirit."

Pema Chodron, a notable author and teacher in the Shambhala Buddhist lineage, says that in life we can't eliminate what we fear from showing up and just get the goodies: so we can cultivate equanimity or non-attachment instead of liking and disliking things. She says "pain is always a sign that we are holding onto something," and suggests that we begin to notice our aversions and cravings, asking, "What repels and attracts me?" If we stop judging ourselves and just get curious, we may have the space to make a different choice.

Another good question to ask ourselves is, "How do I cheer myself up?" Do you need something external in order to be happy? Why?

I thought about this. I don't watch television much at all but I do like comfort foods sometimes. I love writing and reading so sometimes that's a comfort and escape. I love date nights and romance with my husband which is definitely an escape from reality at times. To me, it's good to have strategies to cheer ourselves up but we also can become awake to whether those strategies also sabotage us.

Ask yourself what you do to cheer yourself up. What are you particularly compelled by? Once you identify this, just notice how and when it shows up, and then see if you can't try and let go of it a little and find peace anyway.

Pema Chodron says that the Dalai Lama tells a story about trying to catch mice when he was a boy in Tibet. He didn't try and hurt the mice but he wanted to outsmart them. He called them "models of enlightened conduct" because these mice figured out what they needed to do for themselves to refrain from short-term pleasure (the cheese) in order to have the long-term pleasure of living. He says that we humans should follow their example.

MONKEY JAR ATTACHMENT EXERCISE

Think about what monkey jar attachments come up in relation to cancer. Are you having trouble eating good foods? Keeping your treatment appointments? Are you attached to the idea of not having cancer (meaning you have not yet accepted your diagnosis and path)? Are you attached to the idea of not dying? Where might you let go and surrender?

Meditation

The mind's natural condition is peace. Then a thought enters, you believe it, and peace seems to disappear.

BYRON KATIE

Meditation is said to quiet the chatter of the mind so that you can connect with your Higher Self. It is supposed to be especially helpful in dealing with the stress of cancer. According to an article in Cure magazine by Don Vaughn called "The Calming Effect," a therapist named Elaine Rosenbaum used mindfulness meditation to reduce stress in cancer patients. She says that cancer is one of the most stressful diagnoses a person can endure. It brings anxiety about diagnosis and recurrence. Evidence suggests that the body's numerous chemical responses to stress may affect cancer growth and also influence how we cope with treatment.

Mindfulness meditation is associated with lowered activation of the amygdala, an area of the brain associated with the fear and stress response. There are approximately 125 open trials on mindfulness currently being funded by the National Institutes of Health (NIH). In 2011, in an international complementary medicine journal, researchers analyzed 6 reviews and 19 original papers and found that mindfulness meditation can reduce distress and improve mood and quality of life for cancer patients. Meditation has been used in the treatment of a variety of medical conditions, such as high blood pressure, anxiety, and intestinal problems, as well as cancer.

Also, deep breathing while you meditate is important because when you are stressed, your body becomes a waste dump and breathing releases those toxins. So, meditation can relax you and calm your mental and emotional state while deep breathing clears you of toxins on the body level.

Jon Kabat Zinn, an author and meditator teaches a mindfulness meditation class at a hospital. It's a 2-hour weekly class that lasts for a 6-week period. The participants do 45 minutes of daily meditation and homework and there's also an 8-hour silent retreat. He teaches people to be mindful during daily activities. Over many years of teaching these classes, Zinn has found that patients experience a 25% reduction of the number of symptoms and 32% reduction of illness-associated symptomology such as anger, anxiety, and depression. Their stress hardiness increased 6% and their sense of oneness, belonging, and connectedness increased as well. Follow-up studies revealed that 4 years after taking the class, 98% were still practicing something they had learned in the program. Kabat Zinn says the most significant benefit for patients from mindfulness meditation is learning they aren't their thoughts or their pain or suffering. He even teaches med students to meditate, in attempt to help them reduce stress and increase empathy.

In 1966 Maharishi was a spiritual guru who developed Transcendental Meditation to bring enlightenment worldwide. In a study he did, meditators had a mantra and practiced twice a day for 20 minutes, which refined the nervous system and mind, increased intelligence, creativity and fulfillment. Studies have shown that subjects studying this meditation technique found physiological and psychological integration and their sense of well-being significantly increased.

If you've never meditated this could be a great time to begin. I've included some guided meditations in the resource section. It can be easier to start with the structure of a guided meditation. You can also join a meditation group in your area.

Most of the time during my cancer treatments I did a daily 10-minute guided meditation from Christopher that I kept on my iPhone. I found that just that short amount of time meditating would calm me, my energy level was higher and my thoughts more positive, and I was more present and open. Christopher suggested that the next time I was stressed and wanted to reach for the M&Ms, I should take ten minutes to listen to my iPhone meditation first. Then if I still wanted the candies, I could go ahead and eat some. I call this the Zen diet! When I remembered to do this it often worked!

Limiting Beliefs

Reexamine all you've been told.
Dismiss what insults your soul.

Walt Whitman

Sometimes we have beliefs that don't serve us or make us happy. In fact, they limit us from seeing or experiencing healing possibilities. For example, the belief that "I must have cancer because I deserve to be punished," or "I have cancer because I did something bad." Such statements are not only false, but they trigger guilt and shame, which are very low thought/feeling vibrations and will not help on your healing path. We are trying to increase our love and gratitude vibrations throughout this journey instead. One of the best things you can do for yourself is to increase your thoughts and feelings of love and gratitude, which are high-energy vibrations. You can begin by noticing every time you make negative statements or have these negative thoughts, and then challenge yourself to immediately say something positive instead.

You may be thinking, "Well cancer *is* a bad thing. How does she want me to have positive thoughts and beliefs about that?"

This is a good question but it is possible, and context is king. I explained in the beginning how having a spiritual context for cancer enabled me to learn, grow and contribute from this experience, instead of feeling victim to it.

The exercise here is to observe your mind without judgment. Just watch the ups and downs and notice what comes up and whether it is sourced from love or from fear. When you are on a train of thought that you don't like, you can always choose to get off.

Penny Pierce, author of *Frequency* says, "Whenever you unlabel something or pull your invested energy out of a fixed idea or definition, you dissolve another shadow and more diamond light flows through your life." You can do this with cancer.

In *Healing and Recovery*, Dr. David Hawkins speaks about how the mind creates illness. He reports that he had 20 illnesses, including a duodenal ulcer, colitis, hemorrhage diverticulitis, migraines, Reynaud's disease, gout, high uric acid level, severe hypoglycemia, pancreatitis, gallbladder attacks, a pilonidal cystic tumor, inguinal hernia and more. He says he cured them all within 2 years by changing his beliefs. Now before I go any further, let me just say that I am not advising you stop any medical treatment or even suggesting that you believe this. I am relaying his story because it cannot hurt to work with your belief system while you progress with your standard medical treatment. Hawkins says you should refuse to buy into the collective beliefs about various diseases and symptoms.

Okay, so according to Dr. David Hawkins our mind directs our body since it is more powerful. He would release any symptoms and cancel them by saying, *"I cancel my belief in duodenal ulcers. I'm subject only to that which I hold in mind. I am an infinite being and in truth, I am not subject to that. That is a fact."*

The idea is that if you say this and replace "duodenal ulcer" with "breast cancer" and really mean it, your body may respond to your new belief. Hawkins would cancel the belief in any symptom or illness, surrender to divine will, forgive himself for any limitations and stop attacking himself.

Again, you can choose to try this technique or not, but I am not recommending you stop medical treatment.

On a more humorous note about your beliefs, Bertrand Russell says, "I would never die for my beliefs because I might be wrong!"

EXERCISE IN YOUR LIMITING BELIEFS

Take your journal and write down any limiting beliefs that will put you into fear and stop you from moving forward in love. Then challenge them and shift to a more positive, productive belief. For example:

"Only negative people get cancer."
"My life is over."
"I'm going to die."
"I can't make it through all this treatment."
"I will be ugly bald."
"I'm being punished."
"God doesn't love me."
"No one will care if I am gone."

The truth is that each of us has had similar despairing thoughts, even if they were fleeting. But what makes a difference to your healing path is if such thoughts are a reflection of your beliefs, rather than just a moment of overwhelm. Take some time to challenge any negative beliefs you might be harboring. For example, "My life is over." Yes, your life as you knew it will never be the same again, for you have been touched by cancer. But there are hundreds of thousands of cancer survivors telling their story about how having and surviving cancer changed their lives in significant ways for the better. That while difficult, scary, painful and undesired, cancer pushed them deeper into themselves, into noticing and appreciating life in the ways that really matter, into being better parents or spouses, or bosses, or stewards for humanity. You too can choose to view cancer as an invitation to spiritual growth and to an even more powerful life.

For me, having cancer revealed to me that I wanted to leave a legacy of writing and publishing 22 books, and four books were written during my cancer treatment. I also shifted some lifestyle habits and made a much deeper connection with my Higher Self and Spirit. This could be your best year yet. Don't waste any more time imprisoned by your limiting beliefs!

Stop Labeling Yourself a Victim

As we release 'victimhood', we can bid farewell to our victimizers.

MICHAEL MIRDAD

When something challenging happens to us, it is normal to ask, "Why me?" and to feel like a victim. You do not want to go too far down this road because you probably won't get an answer and either way, this *is* happening so you can choose to accept it or bemoan your current existence.

This isn't happening to you because you were bad or because you are being punished. It isn't being done "to you." It is working its way *through* you. And you can choose to become a channel of love, strength, growth and grace, and be a leader down *that* path, or you can be a victim, a person who feels powerless to the bad things that they feel are being unfairly *foisted* upon them. The choice is yours.

How does being a "victim" sound to your soul? How does that word feel in your body? Does this sound like your true self? Yet it is easy to slip into this identity description when you are tired, in pain, or feeling unloved. It's important to notice when you do this and choose again.

You can speak lovingly to yourself and remind yourself that you are a brave leader on an unmarked path and your mission is to learn more. You can remind yourself that you are a child of God and as such you are *always* loved and powerful, no matter the circumstances.

As a psychologist I've found that we "live into" our identity descriptions, so it is powerful how you frame your situation and your role in it. If you think you are powerless and helpless your body can respond to this, and it will react according to those messages and just give up. Ask yourself: How can you become the heroine in this story? What are the learning points in this life chapter?

It's also important to remember that into every life some rain (and pain) will fall. So it may feel as though you were singled out but all people have their trials to bear. This is why many people recommend that the quickest way to get through challenges is to help those who are even less fortunate then you. This will remind you of your power and blessings and help you to alleviate the suffering of others, which is good for them *and* for you.

Past-Present-Future Dichotomy

Do not bring with you one thought the past has taught, nor one belief you ever learned before from anything . . . come with wholly empty hands unto your God.

A Course in Miracles

Fearful thoughts are often not based in reality because they are not based in the present. Often we are thinking about something from the past or something we fear will happen in the future. For example, if you've been diagnosed with cancer you may think about what your doctor told you in the past or you may worry about cancer returning in the future. When we are dwelling in the past or the future we are draining our energy into something we can do nothing about.

So cancer can be an opportunity to discern and practice this three-fold dichotomy and choose to be PRESENT. When your next fearful thought pops up, ask yourself "Is this from the past, present, or future?" If it is happening in your future (like a possible symptom or the fear of death) then it may not happen at all. If it is past-based, then it's over and you are only reliving it in fantasy. Return to what is happening now. Do not feed your fear. If it is something bothering you in the present then you can address it, take action, and then be done with it.

Frustrations & Adaptability

The dominant illusion is that once we vanquish the next enemy, overcome the next obstacle, get over the next hill, life will be secure, free of problems, perfect. In real life, on the other hand, I have yet to meet a person who has said, for any length of time, 'I'm done!'

Arianna Huffington

I am clear that part of this cancer path for me was learning to be more adaptable. As a therapist by profession I was wed to structure, planning, responsibility, and reliability. When I was diagnosed, most of my well laid out plans went out the window and I had to (begrudgingly at first) surrender to the universe more and be open to the lessons being offered.

I described how I had to change hospitals mid-treatment, how "You Can Thrive" started charging for classes so I had to stop going there, how I had to change my schedule, and that I lost my hair. Then my cancer yoga class changed times and locations on Tuesdays so I couldn't go to that anymore. My one close cancer friend Jen went to stay at her mom's house in Washington DC (after having her chemo in NY) so I didn't get to see her too much either. I was happy for her because this was in her best interest, but it just seemed like one more personal adaptation I made during my treatment.

I began to understand that mentally and spiritually, adaptation is learning to surrender your attachment to how things should be, and learning to be content with the present, no matter what. Challenges also make you adept at problem-solving. It is recommended that when faced with a challenge you come up with 7 alternative possibilities to resolve that challenge. For example, when my yoga class switched time and locations, I could: use a yoga video instead, change my client schedule and attend the yoga class at its new time, write my teacher Tari and ask her to make it later, take another yoga class in the city, use that time for something else productive like writing my book, get a massage, or something else self-care related. This is an example of a brainstorming process and how it opens up options when it seems like a door has closed. Life can be unpredictable, so it helps to learn to be adaptable and flow with it.

In *Frequency* Penny Pierce says, "A problem is pointing your attention to an experience you need to have . . . try relaxing into the situation to see what your soul wants you to notice." She also says, "It is your materialized shadows that you interpret as problems, and it is in clearing them that you learn life lessons."

Ask yourself how cancer has made you more adaptable. Where have you learned to bend instead of break?

Tolerations

Human beings tolerate what they understand
they have to tolerate.

Jane Rule

In my coaching program we did a "Tolerations exercise" where we made a list of 100 things we "tolerate" in our life. The list could include anything that seems less than ideal: for example, if your coat was missing a button, if you hadn't repotted a plant, changed a light bulb, or had been tolerating disrespect from a friend. If you do a "tolerations inventory," you will be surprised by how many things you are tolerating. The idea behind this inventory or exercise is that when you discover and address these tolerations, you end up with more available energy. So, for example, when you finally sew on that button that has been missing from your favorite shirt, or get a billing person to improve your practice or order your groceries online to streamline your meals, in the long run you will free up that mental energy of holding on to this little thing that needing attending to, allowing space for other, more significant thoughts to come in. You may also save yourself emotional energy because it drains you to feel guilty or to sit in situations that are not aligned with your values or wishes.

Christopher Dilts pointed this out to me one day when we were discussing my nanny. I had been saying that the nanny was good with the kids and responsible, and things were "okay," but she and I were not in agreement about their diet and meals, even though I went over this when I hired a nanny. And although I was disturbed by this, I explained that I also felt the kids had enough disruption in their routines due to the cancer, and I did not want to subject them by finding a different nanny at this time. He replied that her energy caused an energetic dissonance for me, and this undermined what I was trying to create, which was familial health and a team of people who would row together.

He stressed that this was my home and I had attracted her at one level of consciousness, but I had grown and now I deserved even more support and should not settle. He said my kids' habits would be harder to change later, and emphasized that I deserved someone loving who would say, "You just had chemotherapy, do you want some vegetable juice?" or who would offer to help unload the groceries or find other ways to show her support. He said, "You deserve someone who will listen to you, honor you, and respect you. Imagine holding your home as a positive vision and protecting it from negative energy." I was relieved to hear this from someone else, because I sensed it as true within my inner being. I resolved to take an overall look at where I was holding or giving away my power in our home, once my treatment was finished. He suggested I visualize the help of my angels in attracting a very loving nanny, one who supports me and my kids, and who mirrors my current level of consciousness. Or, to be able to strike an agreement around food and cooking with my current nanny going forward.

So ask yourself, "What are you tolerating in your life that isn't respectful or supportive of you?" Don't overlook the little things. Just like little destructive habits, they add up. And, especially now, while going through cancer treatment or in recovery, you'll need your energy to stay strong and positive. It helps to begin to plug any drains and to build a strong team, even after treatment is over.

EXERCISE FOR TOLERATIONS

Make a list in your journal of 100 things you've been tolerating in your life (big and small). Then go through the list, and one-by-one take care of the intolerance! Write down how you feel as your energy returns to you and you are aligned with your soul.

Contending with the Unknown

Comparing what happened to what you think should have happened is war with God.

BYRON KATIE

If you are a planner, it's hard to deal with the unknown and to accept the lack of things that you can control. This lack of control can often affect your mental and physical health.

Confidence is the ability to handle a situation and this feeling has a positive effect on health. In one experiment, two white rats were put in cages next to each other. Both rats got an electric shock simultaneously but one rat had a lever and could push it to stop the shock. The other had no lever. They received the same shock but only one rat could control it. The rat with no control got stomach ulcers: when both rats were then injected with cancer cells, the tumors spread more rapidly in the rat without control.

In another study by Dr. Arthur Schmale and Dr. Howard Ker, they surveyed 51 women who had taken a test to determine if they had cervical cancer, before their results were given. Sixty-one percent of the women who felt that they had little control over their lives had cancer, but only 24% of women who felt in control of their lives had cancer.

We know that having control feels good and affects better outcomes in our physical health, but what do we do when there's only so much we can control?

For me the answer has been two-fold: learning to relax more into the unknown, and figuring out what I *can* control and shape in my life, and then doing that. So, for "learning to let go" this book offers tools such as meditation, adopting a spiritual perspective, deep breathing and developing trust, and faith in a Higher power and purpose. For learning what you *can* control, you can affect your mental state, manage your emotions, attitude, lifestyle, consciousness and context. That is why this section is so important because the things you do to have mental clarity and a great attitude will always be in your control. I will give you some tips that helped me, as we progress.

In *You're Not Going Crazy . . . You're Just Waking Up!* Michael Miradad says that we need to go through a process of upheaval in order to become more aligned with Spirit in our lives instead of ego. He says the more attached we are to controlling our lives and others around us, the more disoriented we will feel when that control is suddenly gone. And Carolyn Myss suggests that we can unplug our circuits from our need for our lives to follow a linear agenda and live in spontaneity of divine order where all events lead to our divine empowerment. She says as you transform, you unplug from human justice and surrender to divine justice, trusting that things happen for a reason.

In Michelle Whitedove's book, *She Talks with Angels,* she explains The Law of NonResistance, saying that as long as we resist a situation it will remain with us. When we walk through our fears and face that situation, it no longer has power over us.

So, will you resist having cancer or will you choose to surrender to this journey?

Humor

The human race has one really effective weapon,
and that is laughter.

Mark Twain

Humor often helps cancer patients by combating fear, comforting them, making them happy, reducing their pain, and boosting their immune system. A study published in the Journal of Holistic Nursing showed that humor very definitely diminished pain. Dave Traynor, M.Ed, director of health education at Natchaug Hospital in Mansfield Center, Connecticut in "American Fitness" reports: "After surgery, patients were told one-liners prior to administration of potentially painful medication. The patients exposed to humor perceived less pain as compared to patients who didn't receive humor stimuli."

In 2006, researchers led by Lee Berk and Stanley A. Tan at Loma Linda University in California, found that two hormones, beta-endorphins (which alleviate depression) and human growth hormone (HGH, which helps with immunity) increased by 27 and 87 percent respectively when volunteers anticipated watching a humorous video. Simply *anticipating* laughter boosted health-protecting hormones and chemicals.

The same research team conducted a similar study recently to see if the anticipation of laughter that was shown to boost immune systems could also reduce the levels of three stress hormones: cortisol, epinephrine and dopac. They studied 16 fasting males, who were assigned to either the control group or the experiment group (those anticipating a humorous event). Blood levels showed that the stress hormones were reduced 39, 70, and 38 percent respectively. Therefore, researchers concluded that anticipating a positive event can reduce detrimental stress hormones.

A study at Arkansas Tech University showed that concentrations of immunoglobulin A were increased after 21 fifth graders participated in a humor program. Laughter increased their ability to fight viruses and foreign cells. I think someone should create a book of related jokes for cancer patients to take to chemo treatments with them!

The fellow patients I encountered in the waiting rooms usually had a good sense of humor. One woman had been waiting a long time to see her radiologist. He came to get her and was standing there waiting as she gathered all her books and put things together. She looked up and said to him, "I think it's nice once in a while that you are waiting for me!" (This is one of those times when it's helpful if doctors have a sense of humor too!)

My neighbor's sister got thyroid cancer and she decided to have a laughing party. She invited her girlfriends over to tell jokes, laugh, and watch funny movies. Norman Cousins experienced years of prolonged pain from a serious illness and claims to have cured himself with a self-invented regimen of laughter and vitamins. In his 1979 book, *Anatomy of an Illness*, he describes how watching comedic movies helped him recover.

Over the years, researchers have conducted studies to explore the impact of laughter on health. After evaluating participants before and after a humorous event studies revealed that episodes of laughter reduces pain, decreases stress-related hormones and boosts the immune system in participants.

Donna Eden says, "Studies of antibody production have shown that the stronger the person's sense of humor, the more resistant that person's immune system will be to stress . . . Humor jump-starts the radiant currents."

So, laugh it up! Make cancer serious fun. Find ways to laugh, to joke about your situation, and to improve your mood. Laughter just makes us feel good and helps us to lighten up. This allows us to walk that difficult path with a lighter step. It seems silly to waste a day without laughing. As E.E. Cummings once wrote, "The most wasted of all days is one without laughter," and as the Bible says in Proverbs 12:22, "A cheerful heart is good medicine."

The Nature of Habits & Addictions

Humanity I love you because when you're hard up you pawn your intelligence to buy a drink.

E.E. CUMMINGS

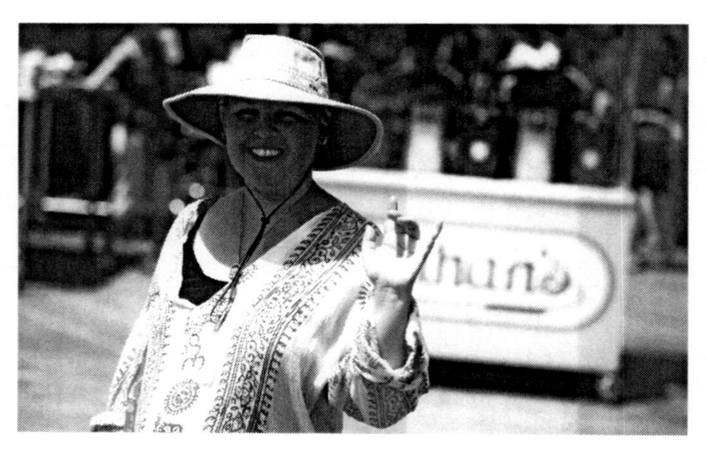

ME SAYING GOODBYE TO THE *NATHAN'S* BY MY HOUSE!

Habits are hard to break. Our behavior forms neural networks in the brain. We form habits through repetitive behaviors and thoughts. These lifestyle habits have a great effect on our health, for better or worse.

One study with astronauts determined that it took 30 days to develop a habit. In this study, astronauts were given goggles to make them see upside down, so that they could practice living that way for their time in space. At first they bumped into things and it was a big adjustment, but as they kept wearing these goggles they discovered something interesting: their brain turned things right side up! But this took 30 days. If they took off those goggles even for a few hours at a time before those 30 days, their brain didn't make this switch! So, it's important to give change time and be consistent.

Dr. David Hawkins developed a "Map of Consciousness," that uses a muscle-testing technique called Applied Kinesiology to document the nonlinear, spiritual realm. Each level of consciousness coincides with human behaviors and perceptions about life and God and represents a corresponding attractor field. The numbers on the scale represent logarithmic calibrations and their significance lies in the relationship of one number to another. This scale ranges from 1 to 1000.

Dr. Hawkins suggests that (according to his Map of Consciousness) the emotion of desire "calibrates" at level 125 and anything under that potentiates illness. He says this lower range represents a negative energy field of consciousness because it is the field of addictions, which can become obsessions and compulsions, and when you are at level 125, happiness is seen as external to you.

We can know all this but changes are still hard to make since we are creatures of habit. We usually make them when we are emotionally ready, unless something like cancer comes along and makes us get ready NOW!

I never thought of myself as having addictions. I didn't do drugs, smoke cigarettes, I'd never been on any type of psychotropic medication or other medications, I rarely drank alcohol and I didn't even like coffee! I ate reasonably well (or so I thought) although I still had 30 extra pounds from my second pregnancy. I did enjoy my diet coke, but only once or twice a month.

Yet as my path narrowed and became more healthy, I noticed I was really struggling to completely eliminate carbs, sugar, and soda, and so I realized I did indeed have an addiction. One psychological definition of addiction is that it acts as a need for something outside of yourself in order to feel okay. Carolyn Myss defines addiction in a more spiritual context and that really stuck with me. She says that when your mind and heart are at war and you can't command your Spirit, this energy comes out of your cell tissue. I needed my power now and my vision had become more attuned and microscopic. I was now thinking of my food choices not in terms of "shoulds" or diets but in terms of energy and where I was losing power to live my fullest life.

Gandhi suggested that we are most powerful when our thoughts, feelings, and actions are aligned. He said, "Happiness is when what you think, what you say and what you do are in harmony . . . Always aim at complete harmony of thought and word and deed." This is easier said than done, but I can see the importance in it for gaining personal power. It takes dedication and practice. Gandhi also said, "An ounce of practice is worth more than tons of preaching . . . My life is my message." For us to have that type of congruence and inner power we need to look at where we are inconsistent and imbalanced. My diet and self-care were now in my face, in a more clear and spiritually focused way than ever!

Researchers recently determined that refined sugar is actually more addictive than cocaine! In a recent study rats were given a choice between sugar water and cocaine, and 94% chose sugar! Even the rats that had previously been addicted to cocaine switched to sugar once they were given the option. Our foods are full of sugar today and most of us were raised to love sugar cereals, drinks, and sugary snacks, so it has unconsciously become a societal addiction or habit.

If sugar is one of your favorite food groups, it can be helpful to think of sweet things you can have often, like sugar free Jell-O, brownie Quest bars, fruit or healthy snack bars. You can even make your own smoothies or fruit sorbet! Go to www.myhealthmaster.com and click on sorbet and ice cream recipes. They have great recipes for cherry sorbet, strawberry gelato, pineapple and wheatgrass sorbet, peanut butter ice cream and even chocolate chip ice cream which is healthier and you can make easily and quickly at home. You can use almond milk, Stevia, real fruit and organic dark chocolate chips, if you have to! If you are out and want a snack, health food stores offer GoRaw treats like the 100% organic *Live Pumpkin bar* or the 100% *Organic Spirulina Energy bar* to munch on. If you really want chocolate, try *Bug Bites* at your health food store. These are organic chocolate squares that have pictures of endangered bugs in them and 10% goes towards that cause so you are doing something good for the environment. Kris Carr's cookbook also has some dessert recipes that are healthier than normal desserts if you really need something sweet.

My sister, Avra, made a few good suggestions about skewing my habits in a better direction. She said that instead of trying to diet and eliminate what I love, I should try to think of it as adding good things in, like fruits and vegetables. She said that before I let myself eat the M&Ms I should eat an apple and then see if I am still hungry and wanting the M&Ms. That seemed do-able. Also, she noted that my kids were developing the habits of loving sweets too. My husband would feed them Eddie's ice cream as a reward when they ate all of their dinner, and I would sometimes bring them lollipops after work. They loved surprises like that and would be so happy to have their treats—but clearly we were passing on the sugar addiction! My sister suggested I create rituals around grapes and apples so they would develop positive loving associations to foods that are good for them instead. This conversation made me realize the lasting implications of simple things like the food we all choose to eat. It made me sad to think of my children struggling later in life with weight or health concerns, and I wanted them to form good foundational habits. I began to see how the body, mind, and emotions and spirit are all connected.

OK, so here's an honest appraisal of what I was able to shift right away, and where I am still stumbling.

Changes I've Made:

1. I largely gave up diet coke after drinking it for years to stay awake.

2. I hated water and started drinking more immediately but I forget to number them and to drink 8 a day. I'm lucky if I am drinking 4!

3. I like walking by the beach and meditating at least 4 days a week, so this change was pretty easy. It helps to enjoy something!

4. I do eat more veggies and gave up most pasta, pizza and baked goods. Occasionally I splurge but I still eat some cereal, Ezekiel bread, rice and quinoa!

5. I started listening to more inspirational music and meditations to raise my vibration.

6. I went to my cancer yoga class weekly until it changed times during my fifth chemo. After that I walked for 30 minutes on the beach many mornings.

7. I gave up alcohol but that was easy because I did not drink much anyway.

Things I Still Struggle With:

1. **Not Using the Microwave.** maybe it's because I'm lazy, rushed, and on the run or that I don't cook but often I still end up nuking things for a few minutes and I'm not sure how bad this radiation is for me, with the breast cancer.

2. **Working Out.** I had yoga and tai chi DVDs at home but I rarely used them. I made the excuse that my kids ran around the living room so I

couldn't focus, but I could have exercised later at night when the kids are in bed. I recently started doing the treadmill for 40 minutes in the morning four times a week, but that was after treatment.

3. **Sleep.** My social worker at Sloan Kettering hospital said most women with my diagnosis and treatment sleep 10 hours and take naps during the day. I laughed and told her I was lucky if I got 6 hours sleep most working days, because both my kids are up at 6 a.m. and we often got home—and thus to bed—late. Ideally, I'd love to get 8 hours sleep even after this is over but I need a go-to-sleep-by schedule and must stick to it!

4. **Affirmations.** I had Louise Hay affirmations on my iPhone and I tried to listen to them a few days a week, and although my goal was to listen a few times a day, I felt like I was too busy to make that a solid habit/commitment.

5. **Deep breathing.** I am still a shallow breather and I talk fast (NY style). I try to do the 3-part breath exercise for 15 minutes in the morning (which is great), but I think it would be ideal to do this a few times a day so I'd learn to breathe this way automatically. I breathe in and out slowly, focusing on my root chakra, my heart chakra and my crown chakra. This would put me into my parasympathetic nervous system and would create clarity of mind.

6. **Surrendering my Ego.** I think this is getting better but I still drive myself to accomplish things and feel that I have to do everything myself instead of surrendering to a Higher Power and asking for help and doing things more slowly.

I'm sure there are more improvements to be made, like daily green juicing, but for now those are what I'm working on to integrate in my daily life. I am trying to congratulate myself for changes I have made so far and I suggest you do the same. None of us is perfect! We are all works in progress!

Author Sonia Choquette says to chant mantras, like "A-do-nai," three times while focusing on what you want to overcome. Do this several times a day for 30 days. She also suggests that singing Archangel Gabriel's name is good because one of his purposes is to help you break old personal paradigms and trust new ones into expression. She feels that by introducing a higher vibration you fight the contraction and shatter your old pattern.

Louise Hay suggests we say, "I'm willing to release the pattern in my consciousness that contributed to this situation."

Write down the changes you would like to make in your journal and ask for help for the ones that are especially challenging. It may take some time but you can do it.

Deepak Chopra believes that when we do simple things like eating and moving, we can actually change our genes. He cited a recent study showing that when people altered their lifestyle significantly by eating better, exercising more, and practicing meditation, this caused changes affecting 500 genes.

He explains that it is the role of epigenes to trigger a gene to turn on or off. When an epigene is affected by something you do or feel, it won't create new DNA but its behavior can drastically change. Genes only affect you if they are switched on. They have no effect if they're switched off: a gene may turn on and off on a fixed schedule, it may turn on and off depending on that person's behavior and experiences or, a combination of the above, says Chopra. When patients change their lifestyle, the genes associated with cancer, heart-disease, and inflammation were down-regulated or "turned off," whereas protective genes were up-regulated or "turned on." *"How ironic that the two things that medicine thought were fixed, the brain and DNA, turn out to be keys for reinventing the body,"* says Chopra.

Chopra mentions that the power of awareness may be key to switching on a tumor-suppressing gene. He says that tuning your body out is the greatest harm you can do because without clearly communicating with your body, you can't expect cells to respond to your intentions. He says, "When love is replaced by an object, the result is addiction."

Donna Eden describes a "Habit Field," which she says is an organizing field that underlies your energy system and regulates your energies, your physiology, and much of your behavior. She points out that Rupert Sheldrake believed that morphic fields influenced not only biological characteristics but mental activity, behavioral patterns, and social organization. The Habit Field maintains the habits of mind, body, and energy, and it is highly stable energy but that if it shifts, physiological conditions follow. Eden sees the "Habit Field" in the fourth layer of one's aura and noticed that it was affected after she worked with the triple warmer, which controls the body's habits. She says that certain glands and energy systems like the hypothalamous, the spleen, meridians, triple warmer, and the basic grid appear to have a particularly strong influence on habit fields. She feels that energy work is often key in changing habits and recommends using guided imagery to alter your habit field because these techniques impact your neurons and shift the energy patterns in your brain. Repetition increases the strength of any organizing field.

David Feinstein writes in *The Promise of Energy Psychology* that energy therapists shift the dopamine and serotonin imbalances to address habits and addictions. He says that the biochemical signature of a person who is predisposed to addiction includes low levels of serotonin combined with too much dopamine. Dopamine motivates you to obtain food, and ensures safety and procreation. Serotonin is secreted when you are full, safe, and satisfied. There's an inverse relationship between the two. According to Ron Rudin, author of *The Craving Brain*, dopamine sends you the craving to have something. According to Feinstein, energy psychologists stimulate certain acupressure points to increase serotonin levels in the brain. Many have used tapping to treat addiction and break destructive habits like weight gain and smoking. They use it to better serotonin/dopamin balances and to alter stress response patterns.

In *To Heaven and Back: A Doctor's Extraordinary Account of Her Death, Heaven, Angels and Life Again*, Dr. Neale implies there could be a spiritual component to addictions or bad habits. She says, "It seems that God sends us to earth with a deeply-rooted desire to seek meaning and spirituality, and until we satisfy this desire, we experience a void in our souls. Some people fill this void with God, some fill it with material possessions or other worldly desires, and some try not to feel this void by deadening their senses with drugs or alcohol."

I take this to mean that perhaps if we could fill our longing with Spirit, we would not reach for the comfort of food or drugs so much.

So try the Zen diet approach: you can meditate before grabbing comfort foods and notice whether your thoughts are loving or self-sabotaging.

Self-Care & Self Love

You can explore the universe looking for someone more deserving of your love and affection and you won't find that anywhere.

MOLIERE

It seems like self-care should follow the section on habits. You need to know that you are most deserving of your love, no matter what anyone says. Also, if you don't take excellent care of yourself, no one else will—and you won't be able to care for anyone else. But you can know this and not do it! I discovered this quite often on my own cancer path.

Normally we're too busy in everyday life to do too much for ourselves and we just chalk that up to business and responsibilities. But when your life is at stake and you have to do more self-care, you begin to really notice all that gets in your way. Your attention becomes crystallized around why you are not doing what is best for you, when it appears to be so simple.

Healthwise, I was supposed to drink water, eat healthy, walk, and do meditation and deep breathing. I was trying to do this while going to the hospital each day for radiation, spending time with my husband and two kids, working and writing a book. So, if something had to lose out, I noticed it was normally my self-care-which I could do "tomorrow!" But this may be what contributed to this walk down the cancer path in the first place, so I needed to make some changes and understand my mental resistance to choosing other thoughts and habits like a focus on self-care as prominent.

I listened to a Louise Hay tape on cancer that included affirmations, and she spoke about how important it was to be kind to yourself and to never criticize yourself. She said that we should look into the mirror and say, "I love you. I really, really love you," and notice what comes up. Another thing you can say in the mirror is, "I love and accept myself exactly as I am."

I was thinking about this while on the subway, and heard an inner voice say, "I don't have time!" I wondered why everything else, like taking care of everyone else, seemed more worthy of my time. Was this something my parents modeled or that I was taught? However the belief got here, it seemed pretty ingrained. Maybe it came from feeling like I had to contribute and do things in order to feel valuable, but the truth is, as Louise Hay says, "You are loveable because you exist." I can see that for other people, and I guess I can see that about myself, but if I can start saying it to the mirror, maybe I'll believe it more and then I can allow myself to slow down and just "be."

Another resistance in the form of my Gremlin's voice said, "If you follow a spiritual path of happiness, spending 3-4 hours a day on meditation, eating right, and self-care, you won't be making any money, or being successful, or paying all your bills! I think this is a strong fear-based belief that holds me back. Louise Hay says that when you really do great self-care and love yourself that all the other areas of your life just fall into place. I love this idea, but sometimes my childish Gremlin plays the "show me FIRST" game, and doesn't allow me to really have staying power with this new intention of self-love and care.

Louise Hay talks about approving of yourself now, exactly as you are, and she says love is the answer to healing. She says she healed herself of cancer through forgiveness, self-love, and changing her thoughts and diet. I believe this was true for her and I think sometimes cancer can be caused by an emotional issue like resentment or fear, but I don't know if it's always that. Regardless . . . it is always a good idea to increase self-love and forgiveness and to decrease busyness and self-criticism.

Louise Hay is the queen of self-care and self-love. She describes her daily routine in her 80s: She begins her morning by snuggling in her bed and thanking it for a good night's sleep. She tells herself it's a good day. She thanks her body and stretches. She used to do 15 minutes of trampoline but now she stretches instead. She meditates for 30 minutes and asks, "What do I need to know?" Then she makes herself some tea and goes back to bed for some spiritual reading. She takes 2 hours to herself before seeing people. She does positive affirmations around the day's activities and eats a healthy breakfast, usually fruit or fruit juice. For lunch she often eats a large salad and for dinner steamed vegetables and a grain or fish or chicken. When she goes to sleep, she says to herself, "Life loves me." She says, "If people can get hold of their day, they can get hold of their lives."

We can all improve our self-care and self-love a little at a time. By creating our own self-care routines, we make sure to prioritize it.

Organization & Time Management

Dost thou love life, then do not squander time,
for that's the stuff life is made of.

BENJAMIN FRANKLIN

I had been in the habit of telling myself, "I have so much to do and very little time." With the cancer I had even less time, which added more stress. But the cancer also made me aware of this message, so I would challenge it. Chris told me that my level of success came from breathing in the Divine mother in my root chakra. He told me I could be centered and calm because I was more receptive now that my Divine mother was always holding me. As I write this the image makes me smile. My own Gremlin (negative voice) has everything to do with "being busy" and having a monkey-mind. When I'm in the Divine flow things are centered, fun, trusting, inspired, calm and grounded.

Anyway, I thought that I was pretty good at time management, yet ironically, I still did not feel I had much time. I got a lot accomplished but I often had the feeling that there was more to do. Two-thirds of my list would roll over to the next day.

When I was going through chemo I still wanted to work but I created small pockets of time for self-care, treatment, and healing. This felt better. I never thought that was possible until I HAD to do it! So, if you aren't working during your treatment, I encourage you to take as much time as possible for yourself. Write poetry, keep a journal, watch movies, and read books you love. Heck, write a novel! Cancer makes you reconsider your priorities. Write down what you enjoy and what you'd love to learn and accomplish, and get started as much as your health will allow you.

My clients were accommodating when I switched their appointment day so I could take a cancer yoga class on Tuesdays. My husband managed with our kids so that I could walk and meditate an hour in the morning. He would go for his hour-long jog right before me. Grandma took the kids the day I had chemo and weekend days when my husband was working so I could rest and finish this book. Ironically, perhaps I managed time better when I rested some and pushed myself less and was more flexible. My editor Julie relayed a story about the Dalai Lama, asking one of his aides what his schedule was for the upcoming day. The aide told him that his day was very busy, full, lots to do. The Dalai Lama replied that in that case, he would then meditate for 4 hours instead of his usual 2—so he could be in the right frame of mind to attend to all of his obligations. We could learn from him!

You can create a schedule but make room for surprises and allowances for how you feel. Some days you may be nauseous, dizzy, or have bone pain, and plans may have to take a back seat to your body. Chris would say to me, "Divine timing is leading us where we need to be." I began to let the universe lead me as much as I led it; well, it was a closer split anyway. Christopher liked to use the metaphor of a sailboat. He said that if the winds weren't there that day, I shouldn't trim the sails and try to paddle the sail boat. Instead, I should clean the deck, make a meal, or review the chart to use that time wisely but I shouldn't go against weather conditions. I needed to learn how to accept and work with them.

Stepping Stones

So when issues arise, we should see them as
stepping stones not as stumbling blocks.

MICHELLE WHITEDOVE

I remember when I was halfway through my radiation I was so tired and ready to quit! I had done 14 treatments but still had 20 left. To get through it, I imagined 20 stepping stones that could get me to where I wanted to be. I visualized slowly moving through each one, and knew I would come to the end of the path.

What are your stepping stones? You can even draw them out and check them off as you go. Acknowledging your milestones is crucial because sometimes the cancer path can feel endlessly long and directionless!

A tool that some life coaches use is called a Flow Chart. This involves drawing a beginning and end point and a line connecting them. Then they create circles all along that line to fill in the steps in between.

Being able to picture and chart your path and each stepping stone will let you celebrate progress. Try not to get ahead of yourself but always keep the end in sight.

Resources & Help

Good planning requires you to utilize your resources and to delegate, especially when you have cancer and are going through chemotherapy.

The first person to speak about this with is your partner, if you have one. When I was first diagnosed with cancer my husband thought I should continue on as normal. My social worker at Sloan Kettering intended to speak with him, before I switched hospitals because she felt he was being unrealistic about my symptoms and energy level. She recommended that he read a book called *Breast Cancer Husband* (that we never did buy but maybe it would help your spouse!). She told me that she had worked with many women who had my triple negative breast cancer and 70% of them did not work during their treatment for a year, and those who did work part-time would come home and sit on the couch with their tongues hanging out and do nothing with the kids. When I relayed this information to my husband he thought it was ridiculous. He expected things to go on as usual. I hoped they would too, but I wasn't sure how I'd feel and I knew I might need more help.

He seemed willing to help a bit more with the kids. He had a harder time discussing the cancer or giving me extra hugs. But he did get our children up in the morning to change and feed them. This allowed me to lie in bed a little longer and to take a walk on the beach or meditate before going to work. Getting out before it was too hot in the summer would ease my nausea. He needed his jogging time too, so he would do that at 6:30 a.m. and I'd go for my walk at 7:30 a.m., in shifts. He also picked me up from work two days a week so I didn't have to take the subway home for 90 minutes after a long work day. He also came with me to most of my 8 chemo days.

My friends left messages offering to babysit but I didn't take them up on it. It was just nice when they'd visit and take my mind off things. A high school friend, Rachel, came to chemo once to do Reiki on me because she was getting her certification. Another high school friend Jill sent me a video of her making low carb recipes to support me in my new lifestyle, and sent me two books on health and visualization, all the way from California. My high school friend Karen who was a doctor found me a new doctor at Beth Israel after I left Sloan and checked in on me to answer any medical questions. My friend Aida visited and called. It was good to see how different people offered help in their own ways. One thing about getting cancer is you can become more open to help and love. Sometimes it's disappointing when help doesn't come in the ways you think it should and people seem limited, but it's very sweet when it flows to you in unexpected ways.

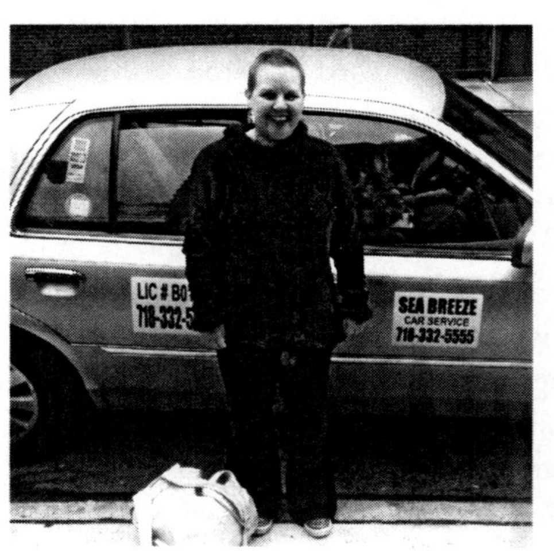

Your energy will eventually come back but you may need extra help, love, and support in the meanwhile so don't be afraid to ask.

Your hospital may offer free resources too. I took a free, 3-session writing class offered by a cancer survivor at Beth Israel. Members of my class were survivors who were also taking free knitting classes, art classes and yoga. Avail yourself of these resources and don't be afraid to ask for help when you need it, and allow others to be helpful.

Money

You're worthy of prosperity.
Your consciousness is the best bank account you can have.

LOUISE HAY

Having cancer often brings up security and money issues. Now that I had cancer, I had to work a bit less. Having my own private psychology practice means I have no vacation or sick days, and since I generally take insurance clients, I don't bring in the higher rates that many psychotherapists do. If I do take days off, I don't bring in any money. Plus, I take my work very seriously. I knew my clients needed me and I was not easily replaced. So, I was committed to working as much as possible throughout my treatment

But this situation made me realize that I should have 4 months living expenses saved for an illness and vacation time. It also made me revisit my fee structure and look at my self-care in terms of how little I charge my clients comparatively with my peers and colleagues. I had to take a hard look at whether I was holding myself back from goals like financial security by disparate beliefs and emotions.

I am still unsure about how to proceed with this. People are more important to me than money, but I know that getting my family on a proper grounding would benefit me, my relationship with my husband, and our kids. The trouble is that neither Ian or I care much about finances, nor are we terrific at managing it. At least we are not in any debt and we are so blessed to have everything we need.

I decided not to make any major business decisions and changes during my treatment. It was enough just to get through that and maintain most of my clients but it did bring my awareness to this important issue for the future, and your experience may evoke similar self-inquiry.

I told Chris that I tend to feel some scarcity about *time*, as well as money. I tell myself that there is not enough time to do everything I need to do. He said, "Well, what would be possible if you allowed your angels to create the belief of having more time to focus on what's important and to let other things remain undone." He said to ask my angels to filter, sort, and prioritize so only my highest potentials came through. So for example, in my spiritual work the angels said that my highest priority was doing my 3-part yoga breathwork, my root/crown/heart meditation, and putting my angelic matrix around me. Chris said that if I practice this it will only take 15 minutes and I can go into it faster and more deeply, like presets on a radio dial. He said I could create the feeling of abundant opportunity, money, and time easily through this practice.

He pointed out that taking classes takes time, and I already have taken all the classes that I need. He said, "Your mind thinks you have to know more but it's about *practicing* what you know. Classes are dangerous for you because your mind thinks that you have to master things and your mind always tells you that you need more. Practice is more important than new wisdom, and you need to practice the basics."

Christopher spoke to me about reclaiming a prosperity consciousness and many other healers write about this as well. Michelle Whitedove wrote in her book, *She Talks with Angels*, that The Law of Prosperity assures that the measure of a person's self-worth and self-love dictates how much they receive.

Similarly, Louise Hay says that abundance and prosperity is about letting yourself accept and feeling you are worthy of prosperity. She says we should imagine an ocean of abundance and notice whether we are holding a thimble or a pipeline. She says, *"Your container is your consciousness. It can always be exchanged for a larger container."*

This is a good exercise: Imagine receiving all good you can receive with open arms and be open to take it in as you would Love.

Of course, we can all also do work to make changes in the money area on a conscious and pragmatic level as well. I decided to give myself a few months to return to normal. At this time I did a balance between accepting a few more insurance patients who called and then saving a certain number of hours to attract full out-of-pocket coaching and psychotherapy clients. I also decided to start a cancer group as a new way to increase my income and share my experience. Over time I plan to transition into full-paying clients and work half-time so I can write more and reach more people, speak to larger groups, and increase my time for self-care. I will create six months living expenses, sick and vacation time in case of another medical scare.

If you work for someone else you may want to consider asking for a promotion or raise or inquiring about the necessary steps to work towards this.

Some people begin a side business from home where they can begin to bring in more income and have a more flexible schedule. There are endless options such as teleclasses, writing, sales, crafts, an organizing business, etcetera.

Once you pay attention to getting this area of your life in order you can find the help you need to increase your resources and security so you have a better foundation should illness or crisis strike again.

Affirmations

I imagine that yes is the only living thing.

EE Cummings

Limiting thoughts are what we say to ourselves out of fear. Affirmations are what we say to ourselves out of love, abundance, and possibility.

I started listening to Louise Hay's affirmations at home or on the subway, but I have to admit that I felt somewhat embarrassed doing this, so at first I only listened to the subliminal version—the side of the DVD that just sounds like elevator music, but has subliminal positive messages embedded in the music. I figured it was still having a positive effect, but no one would know what I was listening to! The other side of her tape is her voice saying things like, "You are loveable just as you are." These positive messages shouldn't feel embarrassing because they're healthy. I started listening to the side with her voice now, so maybe that's progress. Why is it we are embarrassed about saying nice things to ourselves yet we brag aloud about our downfalls and downward comparisons?

Louise Hay says, "Create statements that build you up rather than beat you up." I like that. She says that choosing your words will either help you to eliminate something from your life or will help you to create something new. She tries to think happy thoughts and says she is able to doing this about 75 to 80 percent of the time at this point. She says this practice has made a big difference in how much she enjoys life and the good that now flows into her everyday world.

Doreen Virtue says, "Don't fret repeatedly. Expect repeatedly." She wrote out and recorded her own affirmations and would play them three times a day. They all manifested in her physical world.

I haven't yet recorded my own affirmations in my own voice, but maybe you will. One way to do this is to think of how you want your life to be and to create affirmative sentences in the present. For example:

"My body is radiantly healthy."
"I am peaceful and centered."
"Our finances are abundant and secure."
"Our dreams are coming true in every moment."
"I am an instrument of Divine peace."
"My soul's mission is happening now."
"I am attracted only to healthy food."
"I have a terrific balance between work and play."
"I am making a complete recovery easily and joyfully."

You can think of your own! It is an important step to begin to program positive self-talk because we speak to ourselves non-stop, all day, every day. Author Sonia Choquette says that releasing yourself from criticism is an indication that you are advancing to higher levels of awareness. It's good to view everything through the eyes of love, Spirit, and not your ego, and affirmations are the voice of unconditional love.

In *The Promise of Energy Psychology*, Feinstein suggests that you tap in your affirmations and also visualize what you're affirming. So for example, for the affirmation "I am attracted only to healthy food," you can imagine yourself happily eating fruit and salad while tapping your 8 acupressure points. It may be fun to practice combining some of these tools for greatest success.

Films

The movies we love and admire are to some extent a function of who we are when we see them.

MARY SCHMICH

Movies can be cinema therapy, using imagery, plot, music, etc. for insight, inspiration, emotional release, and change. Sometimes we can see ourselves in the characters or subjects of films. This lets us relate to our issues with more distance and compassion. It can be helpful to gain information from films about cancer. If you love watching movies it can be a fun way to learn and grow on this journey. Some of these films will be inspiring, sad, or painful but they may make you feel less alone.

I recently watched *One a Minute* starring celebrities who had breast cancer, including Olivia Newton-John, Diahann Carrol, Sheryl Crow, Jacqueline Smith, Melissa Ethridge, Lisa Ray and many others who share their experience. You are in good company. Another film I saw was called *Fierce Grace*. In it, Ram Dass discusses how his diagnosis and medical path raised his spiritual consciousness and better helped him serve others. I recently rented *Now is Good* starring Dakota Fanning. Her character is dying and struggling to live her bucket list and make peace with her life and death. What inspiring films have you seen that I could include? See my resource section for a list of inspiring and informative cancer movies.

Teachers & Role Models

A teacher affects eternity; he can never tell
where his influence stops.

HENRY ADAMS

Shamans (Native American healers) say that you are as powerful as your greatest teachers. I tend to think that having wise and loving people in your life is a great way to draw strength, elevate your consciousness, and hasten your Spiritual growth. It's also a great way to keep your mind clear and your wisdom growing. I love to surround myself with great healers and teachers, especially during challenging times.

I find it inspiring to know the stories of people who have walked the path before me—even though each one of us is different. I remember hearing how knowing something is possible can open up your likelihood of doing it. For example, when Olympic runners were training, their coach asked them to visualize completing the mile in record time. One particular athlete who practiced this in his mind went on to do it in real life. What was interesting was that after he broke that record, a number of other athletes broke the records as well, because now they knew it was possible. So, seeing that someone cured themselves of an illness means that this may be something you could do too.

Two women who have been role models for me lately are Louise Hay and Barbara Marx Hubbard. I am almost 42 years old, but I am changing so much and I am realizing that divine timing can surprise us and that it's never too late to be who we want to be.

Louise Hay began much of her transformation in her 40s. In fact, I think she was my age when she attended that class at the Church of Religious Science and three years later taught and became a counselor for them. Later, she was diagnosed with vaginal cancer and cured herself in six months through nutrition, affirmations, psychotherapy, and foot reflexology. She did colonics 3 times a week for the first month and had a diet of mostly vegetables. After 6 months she reports (with doctor confirmation) being cured of cancer. In her 50s she started her own publishing company (and today her book *You Can Heal Your Life* has sold over 3 million copies) and she has helped innumerable people. At 55 she learned how to use the computer and at 60 started her first garden. At 75 she took an art class and now in her 80s she is taking ballroom dancing. Her publishing house has given a platform to many amazing healers and authors.

Another woman named Tao Porchon Lynn spoke at the Newark Peace summit. She still teaches yoga and is learning ballroom dancing in her 90s. My maternal grandmother died at 99 and she still cooked, lived on her own, cleaned, and lived her life. So I know it's possible to have a rich learning path well into the future, god willing.

Barbara Marx Hubbard describes her transformation in her book *Emergence*, which really touched me. She says that she began her shift from ego to essence in her 60s. After 35 years of inner work, the year long process of meditation helped free her of her anxiety, compulsion and fear of failure most of the time. On her 66th birthday she had a big project to write a curriculum and she decided to rise before dawn and spend three hours in silence, alone. She created a space where she felt secure and protected, with soft music, candlelight, flowers and uninterrupted peace. She would sit, "open and empty," and listen to the fire or rain. She said that her temptation was her egoic need to be working (and I could relate to this) but she learned to just let that tugging go by. After she meditated she would write and gain access to her wise inner voice and receive its guidance. She learned to bring her lower selves (and egoic voices) to her Higher self, and over time she could maintain this level of higher consciousness (most of the time). To me, her journey in her 60s and 70s means that it is never too late for any of us to grow, change, be successful and experience a major life transformation. She is one energetic archetype and mentor for me.

There are many ways to find role models and teachers. One that we've already discussed is to creating a healing team. You can have a life coach, a therapist, an angel guy, a massage therapist, a laughter group, etcetera, if it helps you.

Another way is to use technology. You can download CDs from the world's greatest healers onto your iPod or iPhone and listen anytime, anywhere. You can read great books or look on the web for inspiration.

Christopher Dilts told me that a saint once said that 80% of a person's spiritual development comes from observing those around her who are holding higher love vibrations and consciousness and wanting to emulate this. This makes me feel that the more spiritual teachers you have (if they are the good ones) the better.

I did something that inspires me. I made a collage of teachers I like—even though some of them I have never met in person. I have two such collages hanging in my bedroom above my altar. They remind me that there is much healing, love and wisdom in this world. It reminds me there are great teachers who are on the path to enlightenment and we just need to be open and keep learning and listening. Here is a picture of my collage.

I suggest you make a vision of your teachers and mentors who inspire you. Just get some magazines or cut out pictures of teachers you like from their websites. You just need glue sticks, watercolors, scissors and a poster board. Here are my Teacher Visions:

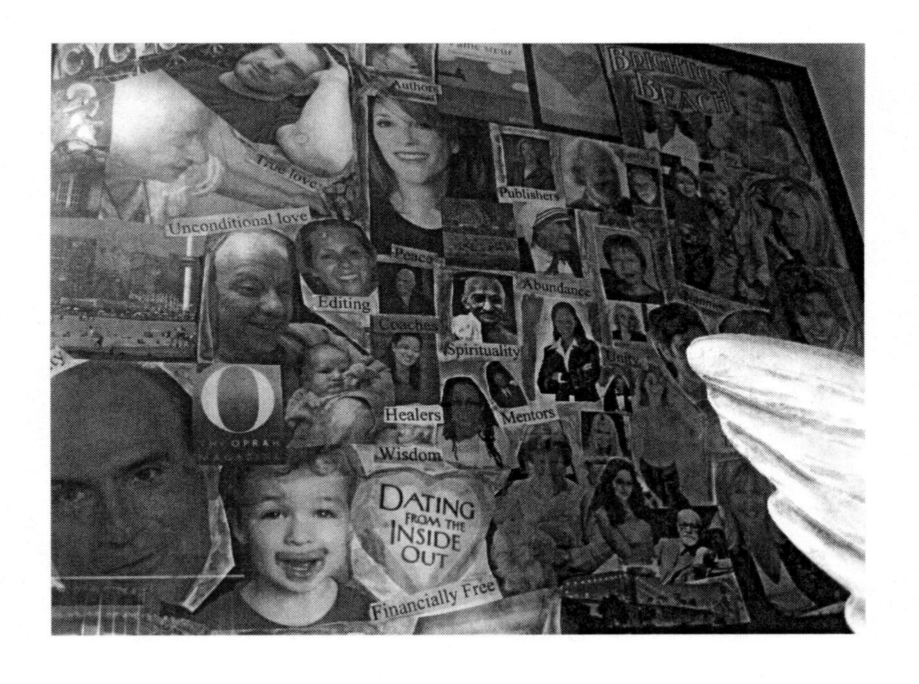

Authors
True love
Unconditional love
Publishers
Peace
Editing
Abundance
Coaches
Spirituality
Unity
Healers
Mentors
Wisdom
DATING FROM THE INSIDE OUT
Financially Free

SECTION III

Emotions

Love makes your soul crawl out
from its hiding place.

ZORA NEALE HURSTON

As a psychologist, when I have worked with people who are sick I have never thought or suggested that their physical illness might have been caused by emotional or spiritual issues. My focus has been to help them cope with their illness and lead a good life in spite of it. This is probably still how I'll proceed in psychotherapy, unless they raise this question themselves.

However, as a patient and healer, when I got breast cancer I wanted to explore all 4 levels of healing and ask a lot of questions, to explore whether the possibility of addressing the emotional level might affect or contribute to my cellular healing. The way I approached most of this was to think, "Well, it couldn't hurt and it might help!"

Many studies have looked at the links between emotions and health. For 2000 years Buddhist thinkers have been aware of the mind's healing capacity. They feel that illness is a result of imbalance in the psychophysical body, produced by conflicting emotions. Studies show that emotional states decrease immune cells. For example, in one study when you weaken the immune system of white rats with repeated electrical shock to the point where their immune system is reduced 80%, they begin to die from different illnesses. This does not happen when their immune system drops only 20-30%.

Howard Friedman at the University of California at Irvine analyzed 100 studies linking people's emotional states to their health. When compared to average people, those who tended to be unusually hostile and angry, very anxious sad, pessimistic and tense, had double risk of getting serious illness, including asthma, chronic headaches, stomach ulcers, heart disease and arthritis. In a study by psychologist Martin Seligman and the National Cancer Institute, cancer patients with "optimistic cognitive styles" had significantly greater survival than those whose styles were less optimistic.

Although we have a range of emotions, many professionals agree that there are 2 basic emotions from which all others derive: love and fear. Cancer can definitely bring up fear but I made the decision to summon as much love and healing into my cells and environment as possible. When I spoke with Christopher about this he reminded me that everything has a vibration, including cancer, and I do not want to attune to that cancer vibration. If I attune to love instead, that is like a bug zapper to the cancer, and love is far more powerful. By the same token, I wanted groups that were supportive but I did not want to join a support group where people just complained about their symptoms or circumstances. To me this vibration would be low and would welcome misery. I preferred to be among people who were trying to learn and grow from their situation and would bring more love into their lives because of it.

In Dr. Hawkins book, *Healing and Recovery*, he says that all negative emotions facilitate illness and all positive emotions tend to cure illness. He says that in most lower energy states (lower vibrations of consciousness) happiness comes from outside the self, and this results in powerlessness, a victim consciousness, and weakness. So the idea is to internalize your power and to find inner happiness and higher levels of calibration in spite of outer circumstances.

Intuitively I agreed with Chris and Dr. Hawkins. It feels proactive to be in a state of love instead of fear as much as possible. But sometimes cancer sucks, and it is okay to cry or feel sorry for yourself when these emotions arise. This allows those emotions to pass through you and to clear, instead of being stifled and getting stuck in your body or psyche.

And clearly, you probably had a life plan and cancer may have derailed it, or at least created a significant detour. I don't want to kid you with all this "love talk." You will probably feel confused and disappointed by a lot of what happens as you go through this process. It's important to be honest about expressing your true feelings. If you need to cry, cry. If you are angry that you have cancer, beat a pillow or talk about it with someone supportive. You are entitled to your feelings and they are normal.

In *Knockout*, Dr. Stephen Sinatra spoke about how crying can be healing for the body. He said the emotional impact of release work on bio-chemicals in the blood like adrenaline, epinephrine, and serum cortisol can be measured in the by-products in the urine. The study showed that participants who had emotional releases had low levels of stress breakdown products in their urine. The men in the study who did not cry or get angry rated high levels of stress hormones, cortisol, and adrenaline.

You can talk to your journal, to God, to friends or to professionals. Some people seek out a social worker, counselor, or therapist so they have their own special time to vent and explore their feelings. Usually your insurance will pay for this and sometimes your hospital will offer this service as part of your treatment team. Check with the social worker there. Other people try group therapy or a support group to vent with like-minded others. Some hospitals even offer free art therapy or writing groups.

Find what works for you as a container to honor your feelings. They need to pass through you energetically so you can move on.

I know it's confusing to find a balance of expressing sadness and anger and being loving and positive. Find what makes sense to you and is most authentic. The idea is to let the sadness and anger pass through you so it can be transformed into self love and acceptance.

Is there an Emotional Meaning of Cancer?

The way is not in the sky. The way is in the heart.

BUDDHA

When I listened to the audio book of Carolyn Myss's *Energy Anatomy* she says that the common ingredient in every dysfunction is an issue of power, and she feels that our bodies are a reflection of what lessons we need to learn and when. She says when the free flow of energy is impeded within the body's energetic system, illness can develop. Negative beliefs, fears and traumas can cause the body to leak energy. I was impressed with her map of our body's energetic system. Although I can't see energy to confirm this for myself on all levels of knowing, intuitively her system rings true to me and I suggest you read her work. I've included it in the Resource section and will sprinkle her wisdom throughout this book as it was a profound resource in my spiritual understanding of illness and how we can become masters of our energy systems and wholeness.

I can't say there is always an underlying emotional meaning to getting breast cancer but some prominent healers suggest that there can be an emotional root so it seems wise to think about it. Do your feelings match some of the underlying causes that some healers identify? For example, Christian Northrup says about breast cancer, "Energy dysfunction often arises when a woman is confused about how to use both her loving (fourth chakra) and her creative (second chakra) energies optimally. The major conflict within women is that most of us still believe that in order to be loved, to receive love, and to guarantee that someone will need us, we must care for loved ones' external physical needs."

Louise L. Hay says, "The breasts represent the mothering principle. When there are problems with the breasts, it usually means we are "over mothering"—either a person, a place, or a thing, or an experience. . . . If cancer is involved, then there is also deep resentment." She says that breast problems have to do with putting everyone else first and refusing to nourish yourself. She says breast cancer can involve deep grief and a feeling of, "What's the use?" She also says that where the breast cancer is located is important. The right side of the body (where mine is) represents giving out, letting go, masculine energy, men and the father. The left side of the body represents receiving, the feminine, and the mother.

I don't know whether the issues of over-caretaking and repressing my full creative expression in these ways were reasons for my illness, but it's important to be willing to plumb your inner depths in the spirit of health and healing.

Gary Zukav discusses how feelings affects the body, saying, "If your thoughts are thoughts that draw low-frequency energy current to you, your physical and emotional attitudes will deteriorate, and emotional or physical disease will follow, whereas thoughts that draw high-frequency energy current to you create physical and emotional health."

What about you? Do any of these aforementioned issues resonate?

On the other hand, if they don't resonate, it may be that they hold no emotional correlation to your experience of breast cancer. In *Prayer is Good Medicine*, Larry Dossey makes a point to say that not all diseases correlate with psychological problems or spiritual failure. He says that many great saints and spiritual mystics died from diseases. Karen Armstrong, in her book *Visions of God*, says that the mystical life itself can seriously damage your mental and physical health! People can reach great spiritual heights and be very loving and still get sick. Ramana Maharshi, an Indian saint, got stomach cancer; the Buddha died of food poisoning; and Saint Teresa of Avila had severe arthritis.

Arianna Huffington makes this point in her book *The Fourth Instinct* when she says that Mother Teresa once told her that people in the West should stop trying to portray her as flawless. Mother Teresa said, *"Spiritual people are not perfect people. They are only imperfect people who have put the Lord first."* I love that quote.

Life is not black and white but we are here to learn. So take this as an opportunity to see if any unresolved feelings could be causing an emotional imbalance. If you address that issue, your body may no longer need to express the imbalance in illness.

Disappointment

You don't develop a muscle without
picking up a heavier weight.

—Marianne Williamson

Disappointment is a low vibration according to Dr. Hawkins, but we don't need anyone else to tell us that it certainly isn't an uplifting feeling! One day I spoke to Chris about how I'd been feeling disappointed by some of the healers in my path (certainly not all of them). I was feeling disappointed in myself because somehow I was attracting these less-than-ideal people and experiences into my life. He said that one reason might be so that I could write about them because millions of other people on the cancer path could be having similar experiences. Sharing my own disappointments might help others to feel less alone and it raised my vibration too.

He also reminded me that no matter diligently I worked to grow and expand, sometimes growth feels painful. He said that when I'm upset I can't receive the guidance from God and my ascended masters and ironically, that's when I need it most. For each of us, it is much easier to receive messages when we're open, trusting, relaxed, and in a vibration of Love. So if you're feeling disappointed, take some deep breaths and open your heart to receive.

Chris suggested that I go to my inner child and look at her thoughts and decisions. Right now she was acting out and not drinking her 8 glasses of water, not exercising, doing 3-part yoga breath, or making green juices, and that's why I was feeling disappointed and discouraged. The inner child was feeling tired and sad, and she felt that people were not being too nice. She wanted to feel comforted, loved and accepted. Chris said to relieve myself of the expectation that it had to come from anyone else and just to strengthen that Divine Love within myself.

He reminded me that our mind and ego says that we should be perfect, but we are more like the tides and sometimes just being able to hold still as the water washes over us is a big accomplishment. If we can hold still the wave will turn the other way soon enough, even as we feel it flowing against us. We just need to hold on to the progress we've made. Sometimes it's easier to go with the flow but standing still and holding your center is impressive when it feels like things are flowing against you.

In *Healing and Recovery*, Dr. Hawkins says that we need to train our minds not to judge, attack, or criticize ourselves or others. He says that within every person is an intrinsic innocence that never dies.

I've found that it is important to never lose sight of the bigger picture or spiritual context for too long, or we fall into despair and lower our vibration, which only reinforces our disappointment. When you can find the spiritual context, you will eventually transition from disappointment back to love. As Martin Luther King once said, *"We must accept finite disappointment but we must never lose infinite hope."*

Think about who and what you are disappointed in, and imagine the tide rolling over you. Can you stay in place and remember Love? Don't be washed away with the negativity, rather, watch and wait until you can get back to a place of centeredness and calm.

Pain & Suffering

Pain is inevitable.
Suffering is optional.

THE DALAI LAMA

We all know that it is rarely the circumstances that make us suffer. It is mostly our reaction to them. Since you are sensitized to physical pain during cancer treatment you can use that experience as an opportunity to sensitize yourself to your emotional pain, and why and how you can deal with it.

When it comes to other people, we know they can sometimes hurt us and it's easy to point the finger. You can take back your power when you learn something from that situation. Byron Katie says, "You are always what you judge us to be in the moment. There's no exception. You are your own suffering. You are your own happiness." Even if it doesn't always feel true, there is something freeing about taking this approach, so you may want to try it next time you have an unpleasant interpersonal situation.

I thought about what different religions teach about suffering. I'm not religious but I was raised a reformed Jew. What I gleaned from my Judaic family about suffering was: complain a lot, be strong, work hard (especially when the going gets tough), use your intelligence to be resourceful and to solve problems, and remember that because you suffer, "you're the chosen one." This last part makes me laugh because I somehow do feel I was "chosen for cancer" or I chose it before incarnation, because it has been a path of learning more about how to help myself and others, and to get closer to God.

In *The Places that Scare You*, Pema Chodron reminds us that life circumstances can harden us so we become increasingly resentful and afraid, or we can let them soften us to make us kinder and more open to what scares us. She explains that *bodhichitta* is our ability to feel the pain that we share with others and our ability to keep our hearts and minds open to suffering without shutting down. A *Bodhisattva* trains in awakening love and courage for oneself and for the welfare of all human beings. She encourages us to ask ourselves what we do when we can't handle what's going on and to examine where we look for strength and where we put our trust.

Consider how you speak when you deal with unkind people. My friend Bradley Hess told me of something Jesus said when he gathered his disciples to give them supernatural power over demons and disease. He sent them to minister to people's needs and to preach the gospel of the kingdom saying, "Behold, I send you forth as sheep in the midst of wolves: be ye therefore wise as serpents and harmless as doves" (Matthew 10:16, KJV). Their serpent-like wisdom would govern the words they spoke as well as the activities they carried out but Jesus wanted them to communicate without hurting the people who heard it—as harmless as doves. This is a difficult balance to be sure, but it's something we can keep in mind lest we lower our vibration by sinking to the level of communication of the person provoking us.

Lastly, we can learn from painful experiences and share that wisdom with others to help them on their way. This increases our compassion and our power. There are two quotes I like that remind us of this message: Viktor Frankl said, "What is to give light must endure burning," and Kenji Miyazoka said, "We must embrace pain and burn it as fuel for our journey."

So, suffering and pain can be mirrors of where we still need to heal and love ourselves more. This can be a way to soften our ego, increase our compassion, nonattachment, and wisdom.

Anger

Out beyond ideas of wrongdoing and right doing
there is a field. I'll meet you there.

RUMI

Dr. David Hawkins says that anger vibrates at a level of 150 on his "Map of Consciousness." This is below the level of truth and power (level 200) and it involves feelings of hate, aggression and antagonism. It's important to recognize that we do not want to remain angry because it keeps us at a low level of consciousness, whether we are aware of it or not.

On the other hand, anger is a normal emotion, so it's good to recognize the injustice you feel and then to move to a higher vibrational state through communication, setting a boundary, or forgiveness. This will ultimately allow you to move from a state of separation and fear into a state or love and unity.

Studies have shown that anger can influence many illnesses. For example, a study by Dr. John Barefoot at the University of North Carolina tested people with heart disease. They were given a psychological test to see how angry they were. The least amount of blockage was found in the least angry group, and those with the most anger had the highest blockage. Researchers at Harvard Medical school found that the single emotion most common in the 2 hours before a serious heart attack was anger.

When the Dalai Lama was having a conversation about anger and the other person was admitting to feeling some anger, he said, "It's fine to have that attitude towards John's faults, because that's authentic, as long as simultaneously you're wishing that John might meet with well-being and be free of suffering."

Of course, most of us aren't the Dalai Lama!

In *The Places that Scare You*, Pema Chodron says that when we are angry we can label the thoughts, "thinking," and let them go. Then we can stay with the energy beneath the anger without acting out or repressing it, and this wakes us up. She recommends that we always meditate on whatever provokes resentment.

I have to say (even while writing this book) that I have not yet tried to meditate while angry but maybe you will and can let me know if it helped you move through it. There will probably be at least a few times that you'll be angry and disappointed during your cancer path so hopefully these words can help.

I would imagine that many people get angry at their cancer and this reaction is normal. I did the first few days but then I was able to shift, thanks primarily to my spiritual context. No one wants cancer. It's annoying and unfair! Yet, on a spiritual and psychological level, "What you resist, persists." So, get angry and let it out but then try and work with cancer to dissolve it instead of remaining at war with it. Staying in anger can polarize you and make you stuck. The idea is to accept cancer and allow it to disappear.

Forgiveness

Non-judgment day is near.

Many people, such as Louise Hay, say that sometimes cancer is caused by resentment. I did not think of myself as a very resentful person. I loved my work and life and didn't think I had an especially tough childhood or trauma in my life.

So is there a relationship between resentment and illness, sometimes? In David Hawkins book, *Transcending the Levels of Consciousness* he writes, "The relinquishing of judgmentalism greatly increases the capacity to love, as does surrendering the wanting of anything from others . . . People are appreciated for who they are . . . Those who have very high levels of consciousness condemn nothing . . . all are one with God, and consequently, that which is intrinsically innocent is within us at all times."

I realized that no matter what the underlying cause, the cancer was an opportunity to transcend tribal thinking, to love myself unconditionally, and even to learn to love people unconditionally who may have wittingly or unwittingly hurt me. It is an opportunity to forgive.

I also started reading a book on auras called *Change Your Aura, Change Your Life*, by Barbara Martin with Dimitri Moralis. In it

Barbara said that our enemies present our biggest opportunities to transcend our inner resentments. She says if someone hates you they transmit an emotional current and you can absorb that current unless you consciously block it. She gives a meditation in her book about how to do this. She also speaks about responding to enemies with love energy. She relayed a story about Mother Teresa who got a lot of resistance from a local Hindu priest. He later became ill and no one would help him, but Mother Teresa treated him with love and nursed him. He asked her forgiveness and became a much more pleasant person. Barbara recommends a meditation in her book and suggests you keep sending your adversaries love so you can move towards that higher level of consciousness and away from antagonism. Although it's challenging, it's under your control to do this.

There was a phenomenon on YouTube my friend Aida told me about, in which a bus driver attendant from Albany was bullied by a group of boys. They taunted her and threatened her until she cried, but she did not strike back. In fact, her self-containment was pretty amazing. One of the perpetrators had posted this video footage to further taunt the attendant, as an act of cruelty, but there was a surprising outpouring of love and sympathy for this lady, so much so that she received $500,000 in donations from strangers and was able to quit her low paying bus attendant job. This was the good part. What I found especially interesting was that people became so enraged that these young boys received death threats. These well-meaning people felt so justified in meeting rage with rage and didn't realize it was the same vibration! This is like parents trying to teach children not to hit by hitting them. It's not easy to stay in a vibration of love when met with hate, but it's worth it. Instead, we sink to the same level and then justify our attitude or behavior through inflated righteousness.

Chris told me a story about his friend and yoga teacher who had died from leukemia. She was a wonderful woman with a big following. For her, the core cause of her leukemia was an unresolved rage at her mother, even after all of her spiritual work. Before she died she healed the relationship with her mom and was able to die in peace, surrounded by her loving family.

So, if you have people to forgive, close your eyes and do a meditation on forgiveness. Picture that person's Higher Self and have a conversation with them. Let them know they hurt you and that you want to release this pain so only love is left. Surround both of you in pink light and watch anything else disappear. Imagine any energetic cording connecting you in pain being dissolved. You can also write a letter to that person stating your feelings and releasing them, and then burn the letter, symbolically releasing yourself from holding any painful or critical energy that is not yours. You are releasing the past and standing in the present with a clean slate.

You can love people because that's who *you* are, regardless of *their* behavior. Marianne Williamson explains that some people try to overcome their own guilt by projecting it onto others. She says we can react by remembering who we are and say, "I love you because it's my true nature to do so."

Pema Chodron says, "The root of compassion, is compassion for oneself," so I don't want to end this section without suggesting that you assess if there is anything you can forgive yourself for. You are not perfect and you are worthy of great compassion for all you are going through!

In *Energy Anatomy* Carolyn Myss says we need to look at our fears and where we think life has been unfair to us—and forgive, in order to heal from cancer and disease. She feels that these fears take away our cellular energy. When our energetic circuits are all plugged in below our waist (in chakras 1, 2, and 3) and are focused on tribal limiting beliefs, criticism, fears, safety, and control, then we need chemical medicine for the physical body to heal. However, Myss says that energetic medicine needs our circuitry to be in the *present* time (chakras 4, 5, 6, and 7) and being able to forgive does this. She points out that before Jesus healed anyone he forgave them and released them from any demons or perceptions that were tormenting them. So, if forgiveness can heal and make you happy and more enlightened, why wouldn't you do it?

Make a list of what you haven't forgiven emotionally and begin there. Remember your innocence and be willing to return to that place of Source.

As *A Course in Miracles* says, "The Ego cannot survive without judgment." Do you want to keep feeding your ego or your Spirit?

Unresolved anger and frustration needs to be forgiven and part of my cancer journey, according to Chris, is to be the lead goose and to break the air resistance for my readers because these things are hard to face. I committed during this cancer treatment to record this journey for myself and others.

Chris said that the most powerful way of dealing with anger is forgiveness and compassion and to use power greater than your own. He offered a prayer from the Angel of Forgiveness:

"Blessed and Beloved Angel of Forgiveness, we call upon you to pour the creamy milk of forgiveness. Pour it within us so we forgive ourselves and over every person, circumstance and experience, for this lifetime, past lifetimes and all lifetimes to come. I call upon your power and strength to allow forgiveness to overflow."

Then let the angels do the work. Keep pouring the milk of forgiveness over that part of you and let love in.

For those of you dealing with difficult people during this especially challenging time, consider this a spiritual test to master the art of remaining "in love" instead of joining them in fear.

In *To Heaven and Back: A Doctor's Extraordinary Account of Her Death, Heaven, Angels and Life Again*, by Dr. Mary Neal, this spinal surgeon recalls speaking to an operating room nurse who had two very difficult supervisors. Neal asked her how she worked for them with such grace and the nurse replied, "I don't work for them . . . I work for God."

Also it doesn't matter what everyone thinks about us, even if they are family and friends. What matters is what we think of ourselves and what God feels about us. And God is unconditionally loving and forgiving so we would do well to emulate this, with ourselves and with others. Try this simple Huna forgiveness practice of saying: "I'm sorry. Please forgive me. I love you."

In *Transcending the Levels of Consciousness*, Dr. David Hawkins explains that relinquishing judgmentalism greatly increases the capacity to love, as does surrendering wants from others. In *Healing and Recovery* he says, "inner peace automatically arises out of our willingness to give up certain positionalties, such as judging others and making them wrong."

Christopher likes the metaphor of a porcupine. He says that someone's quill can touch a place where you are wounded and are in need of healing but once your deeper intuition opens then you can see and understand people better and know their core issues. This reduces their effects on you and you don't take on their issues.

Donna Eden recommends using "The Zip Up Technique" whenever you feel scared, vulnerable, or around toxic energy. She explains that the central meridian is like a radio receiver that channels other people's negative thoughts and energies into you. She describes how pulling your hands up the central meridian draws energy along the meridian line. She says this technique can help you be present with another person in a conflictual situation without their negative energies dragging you down. This might be a good technique to try when you are around toxic people or situations. But after the fact you can always do a forgiveness prayer and let that person and energy go. You can also call upon your angels to surround you with love and light so that only the highest good comes through.

Love Versus Fear

Fear is one of those things that needs to be overcome to reach enlightenment.

Dalai Lama

We have already said that cancer will bring up fear. The question is whether bringing this to consciousness can help you actively transmute it to love. According to Dr. David Hawkins, Jesus Christ said that fear was the last hindrance to overcome and its source is the ego and the failure to relinquish its sovereignty to God. When you really think about it, when you believe in God and heaven completely then there's nothing to fear because you're headed toward a great place. According to his Map of Consciousness, fear is a very low vibration of 100 and it falls below desire and anger. It involves anxiety and withdrawal. In contrast, love begins at level 500 and starts out being conditional and selective but it evolves into a lifestyle and a way of being. Love opens up banks of neurons which await the activation of this energy field and it releases endorphins. Unconditional love vibrates at level 540 and is the energy field of healing, according to Dr. Hawkins.

When you feel fear you can bring in love to allow safety and comfort into your body and raise your level of consciousness. You can do a love meditation to bring love into all your cells. This brings up warm feelings and can open your heart. You can close your eyes and breathe and picture all the things and people that you love in your life. Send them all love and appreciation and say thank you. See yourself and your heart surrounded by green light and let that light move through your whole body. Send love to every cell in your body and thank them for the healing work they are doing and ask that if there are any cells that don't welcome this love and appreciation that they go down into the earth and dissolve like fertilizer. Allow Mother Earth to transmute them into love and growth. See them release and fall away until you are left only with green love and light.

If you have a hard time personalizing this meditation and doing this on your own, then you can order a DVD called *Becoming Love*, by Lita St. James. I've listed it in the Resource section. This meditation can become a daily practice of sending love and blessings to people. You can spend time appreciating everything! You can have all 70 trillion cells in your body attuned to love and appreciation by practicing this ritual. And love is extremely healing.

Dr. Eva Selub, author of *The Love Response*, talks about how the love response causes a series of biochemical reactions that lower blood pressure, heart rate, respiration, and adrenaline levels, allowing balance and well-being. She speaks about reversing stress and fear and programming your biochemistry from negative to positive through a variety of exercises. These exercises are centered around social love, self love, and spiritual love. Dr. Selub was in her residency when she accidentally punctured her finger, exposing herself to the blood of a patient with HIV and hepatitis C. She did an experimental regimen of anti-HIV drugs and was eventually pronounced HIV-free, but she was not the same emotionally, and suffered anxiety attacks. She later quit her job to study alternative medicine and she learned how to give and receive love. As she taught her patients to receive love, they improved. Dr. Selub feels that fear affects every aspect of your mind and body, including brain function, immune system, emotional states, and propensity towards illness. The fear response stimulates the amygdala-hippocampus complex, your emotional center which affects hormones and peptides like cortisol and adrenaline. This can cause your white blood cells to get ready for attack and trigger inflammation. Excessive adrenaline and cortisol production and high levels of insulin are released from the pancreas in response to elevated glucose levels and can lead to diabetes and other metabolic disorders. She says that if you don't use up the energy generated by the Fear Response your body deposits it and stores it in your fat cells instead.

She explains that the immune system is a 24-hour security system that works all day and night. When the immune system becomes overworked, communication between the body and mind is erratic. The brain can lose communication with immune cells and inflammation increases. The adrenals don't produce enough cortisol.

There are trillions of cells in our body, including unhealthy cells like cancer cells. When our immune system functions well, it gets rid of unhealthy cells and creates security walls around them so they don't harm your body. Dr. Selub feels that in a state of love you feel supported and safe. This has a biochemical function creating bonding, attachment and pleasure. The peptides associated with this are endorphins, oxytocin, dopamin, vassopressin and nitric oxide that turn off the fear response and activate relaxation and create a positive psychology. Endorphins can create euphoria and pain relief. Dopamine opposes fear and improves mood and circulation. Science has shown that love and affection stimulate the release of hormones and peptides that improve mood, increase sociability, enhance attachment and turn off the Fear response. Dr. Selub has seen firsthand that individuals who have a positive outlook show improved recovery after surviving acute medical events. She recommends that when you feel bad, you learn to shift from fear to love, and recommends spending at least 20 minutes a day in honoring yourself.

It isn't easy to choose love when fear promises to protect us. But, as Mary Oliver once said, "There are a hundred paths through the world that are easier than loving. But, who wants easier?"

This all sounds good but isn't it normal to fear the "C" word? How can you have a positive orientation towards cancer? Most of us will just be beginning to understand and work towards this. I am explaining my personal understanding throughout this book but I am also trying to include more enlightened teachers and thinkers that inspire me. Christopher Dilts says that we are all on a spiral staircase and we can look a few steps behind us and help those people up. Many teachers help me by their example and I've included some of their words here.

In *A Thousand Names for Joy* Byron Katie writes, "The truth is that until we can love cancer, we can't love God . . . You can't love me until you love your tumor. Every concept that you put onto that tumor, you'll eventually put onto me. The first time I don't give you what you want, or threaten what you believe, you'll put that concept onto me." So Byron Katie probably would love her cancer.

Christopher told me that the great healers healed themselves not by focusing on the diagnosis but on praying for health and bringing themselves into God's love. He offers this as a prayer: *"Hold me in the perfect light and health of God. Take our negative emotions and spiritualize fears so they become holy and sacred. With the Wounded healer, through wounds the love of God flows into us so that we become more loving. Wounds are stepping stones to our own mastery of Spiritual truth, love, and power. Acknowledge your steps on this sacred journey and acknowledge those behind you that you will help to move forward. Eighty percent of a human's spiritual progress comes from examples set by people around them, wanting to emulate them."*

Rumi once said something similar: "The wound is the place where the Light enters you." (I love that!) I think he means that we can use our challenges to help others get through theirs and to connect us more deeply with others and ourselves along the way.

In terms of fear, once we notice our fear and comfort ourselves, we can choose to move towards love. Louise Hay suggests visualizing that our fears are dark clouds and noticing that they get smaller and eventually evaporate.

We can only do shadow work after we establish a foundation of love. Ultimately, our shadow can help us understand where we need to let in light and where we are still wounded. Madame Curie once said, "Nothing in life is to be feared. It is only to be understood." And *A Course in Miracles* reminds us, "If you knew who walks with you, it would be impossible to be afraid."

Carolyn Myss says we need to look at our fears and where we think life has been unfair to us and forgive, in order to heal from cancer and disease because these fears can take away our cellular energy. In *The Path to Love* Deepak Chopra says, "Spiritually the answer to fear is simple: you are already safe."

Jackie Lapin, author of *The Art of Conscious Creation*, points out that fear even affects our global consciousness. She says, "We have relegated our creative visionary power to people who are consciously or unconsciously driven by fear. Fear is the most potent kind of global pollution. What we believe—consciously or subconsciously—determines how we perceive the world and, more importantly, the world itself...It is time we cleanse ourselves of fear and take back the power." Jackie's book is great because it helps us move beyond our personal dramas to envision how we want to create our world. Do we want a world driven by fear (like our current media perpetuates) or by love? We begin by first addressing our individual consciousness.

Acceptance

The only suffering is arguing with what is.

Byron Katie

Part of what we are challenged to do when we get diagnosed with cancer is to accept a reality we did not intend to create. It's a spiritual teaching that contentment does not come from things or situations, it comes from allowing things to be as they are. We can cultivate joy in our attractor field despite the circumstances. Our brain says we can't do it in chemo or when we feel sick but our Spirit and heart knows we can, if we choose this.

Viktor Frankl (*Man's Search For Meaning*) remembers how he could always choose his attitude even in a labor camp during the Holocaust! He was able to talk to trees and imagine a better life. Survivors drew art in the sand to communicate the visions they had for a better life. Their attitude and psyche was their own, no matter what torture their bodies withstood.

Pema Chodron says that its only when we can relax into ourselves without moralizing, harshness and deception that we can let go of harmful patterns, and this begins with acceptance. As Bodhidharma once said, "A Buddha is someone who finds freedom in good fortune and bad."

EXERCISE

Notice when you go into a state of fear and have compassion for yourself. Breathe deeply so that you gain wisdom from your unconditionally loving higher self. Allow that energy to bathe your fear in love and light to become one with your situation.

Gratitude and Appreciation

The litmus test for self-realization is a constant state of gratitude.

—Byron Katie

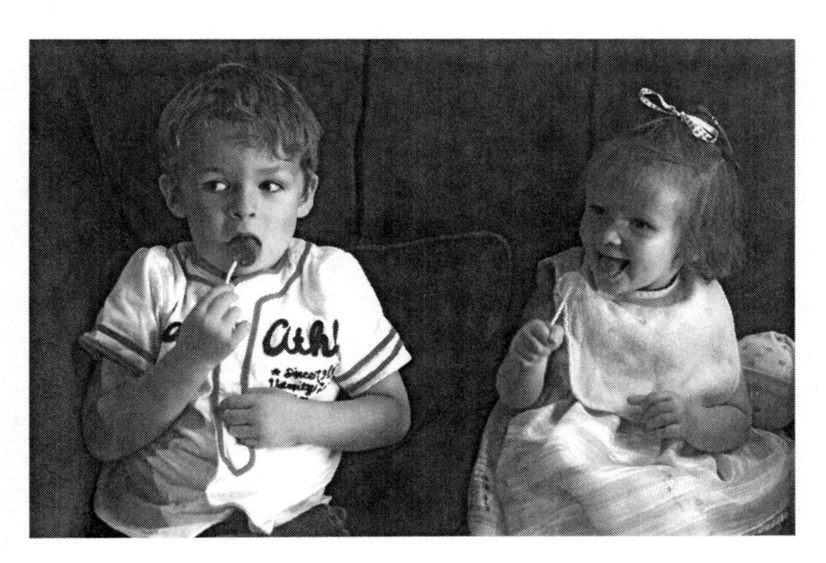

NOBLE AND SERA RELISHING LOLLIPOPS

No one does gratitude and appreciation like kids. They are so in the moment that the level of excitement they exude over a lollipop seems as though they just received an Academy Award. This is something we can reclaim as adults. Think how wonderful life could be if we got so excited about simple things like seeing the sunset, walking on the beach, or going to the playground. My kids have this in spades, so I'm trying to learn from them.

Singer and songwriter Olivia Newton-John (one of my favorites) produced and album called "Grace & Gratitude" that she wrote when she had breast cancer. The chorus for her cover song says, *"Thank you for life. Thank you for everything. I stand here in grace and gratitude and I thank you."* This song always puts me in a very centered happy place.

Music is a powerful way to get in touch with your inner center. For example, Wayne Dyer's daughter has recorded a beautiful version of the song, "Make Me An Instrument of Thy Peace."

Sometimes I like to say thanks for things and people around me. For example, I may say or think while I'm walking the beach:

Thank you for giving me a sexy, spiritual, and loving husband.

Thank you for giving me two most amazing and loveable children.

Thank you for making me a talented, enthusiastic, and creative soul.

Thank you for giving me parents, a step-mom and mother-in-law who lovingly support me through this.

Thank you for allowing me to live in a home I love by an enchanting, healing beach.

. . . and so on.

This may sound arrogant to you but you are a child of God and your spirit loves when you praise your life and put out that energy of love and gratitude. It is powerful. Carolyn Myss says it's the greatest gift to wake up and say that you love your life exactly as it is. She says then you plug into a higher truth that says, *Gratitude is the best attitude.*

This is one way that I knew that something spiritual was awakening in me. Although my body was suffering and weak, on a soul level I felt more love, gratitude and grace than ever before.

Look for opportunities to give thanks. Maybe you have a wonderful doctor or your chemotherapy is now over. Maybe your boss was very supportive and gave you time off. There are always things to appreciate and gratitude raises your energy and sense of vitality.

Joy

The master can't seek fulfillment. She's already filled to the brim!

Byron Katie

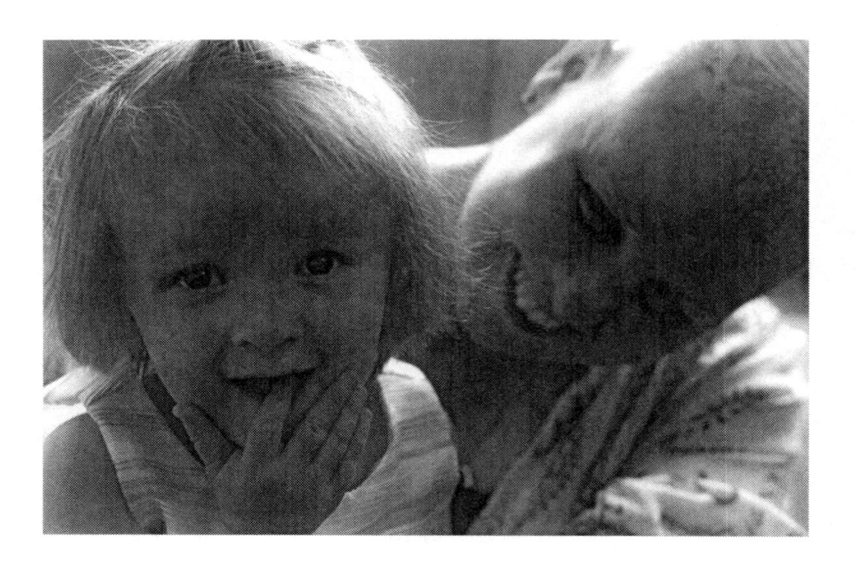

Learning to cultivate joy is huge. According to Baird & Nadel in *Happiness Genes,* microbiologists have discovered a biological basis to human happiness that derives from our inner spiritual world that is different from the Western idea that happiness is external and derives from material things or is action-driven. These authors say that specific genes such as the DRD4 gene and VMAT2 gene are part of the gene pool that promotes a blueprint for intrinsic states of happiness. DNA strands expressed through mindfulness, prayer and altruistic action provide evidence for a neurological basis for spirituality.

Learning to cultivate joy is huge and it may be harder when you are sick. According to a recent study by the Mayo clinic, when you're in poor health you are 70% less likely to be happy than someone in merely good health. But don't worry, we will talk about how to work on this.

In his book, *Transcending the Levels of Consciousness*, Dr. David Hawkins says that research shows that happiness is calibrated with higher levels of consciousness and not externals. He says all psychological studies of happiness confirm that religious or spiritually oriented people are generally happier all the time, no matter what the circumstances (Wellas, 2005). He says that as love becomes increasingly unconditional it begins to expand as inner joy. On his Map of Consciousness, joy is way up there at 540 and it leads to feelings of serenity. It is even higher than love. Perhaps this is because love is often aimed at something, but joy simply is. The Dalai Lama also suggests that the key to happiness is inner peace.

Research scientist Candace Pert says the release of pleasure and intimacy causes the beta endorphin to be released in bonding in simple rodents. Similar receptors in humans reflect back that we are designed for pleasure. Harvard researchers found that the level of cortisol was reduced and natural killer cells increased when people watched funny movies and laughed a lot! Another study looked at 36 women with breast cancer and tumors. After seven years, 24 women had died. Psychological tests showed that the only emotional difference between those who survived and those who died was a sense of joy in their lives. In another study at Harvard, David McClelland found that when people watched a loving film about Mother Teresa there was a brief rise in t-cells and afterwards, if they spent an hour in a loving kindness meditation their t-cells rose for an even longer period.

Dr. Sheldon Cohen did a study where he assessed 193 subjects to determine their level of positive emotions (like happiness, calmness, and liveliness). He exposed them to a virus and found that people who scored low on positive emotions were *3 times more likely* to succumb to the bug.

Researchers at the Arborbanel Mental Health Center in Bat-Yam, Israel, claim emotions affect the immune system's ability to deal with auto immune disorders, cancer, cardiovascular disorder, and HIV. Participants who experienced general well-being had better immune system responses and were less likely to develop disease.

In her book, *Quantum Success*, Sandra Anne Taylor says that love is the most magnetic energy that you can project. It raises your resonant energy and by engaging in the happiness you seek right now, you ensure the future you're looking for.

Write a list of 40 things that bring you joy, to start. Think about your own joy factor *now*, rating it from 0-10 (10 being the highest).

In thinking about the joy in your life, you may have some realizations. For example, I realized that I stopped seeing "having fun" as a priority, or even a large possibility. Instead I was always focused on responsibilities and what I had to do.

I started to think about Archangel Ariel, the angel of joy. Ariel represents love and creativity in our hearts. Adults need joy, not just kids. Christopher told me that when you bring fun into your emotional body it is a brilliant azure blue color. He reminded me that Ariel is the angel of joyful creation and joy was the energy of spring. He also said that joy was absolute poison to cancer. Joy is my natural state, as it is for you as well, so I just needed to give myself permission to return to it.

The other day on my walk I was listening to a Louise Hay affirmation which said, "I allow myself to play every day," and it struck me that this wasn't true in my life. This felt sad. I was whimsical and child-like by nature, so when had I become so serious and "grown-up"? Where was my fun? This is something I'm addressing more going forward. Lucky me, I have two adorable bundles of joy who remind me daily how to have fun.

I think fun for the sake of fun is important (as I just mentioned above) but doing things you are passionate about will also raise your vibration. I love to write so when I began to do this during my cancer experience, it really helped. Milton Erickson, a famous psychiatrist, knew the power of exploring one's passions. One day he met a suicidal woman and asked her what she loved more than anything in the world. She told him it was violets. He told her to give them away and 20 years later she was alive and known by her community as "The Violet lady." So figure out what you are passionate about and do it as a way to contribute and spread your love.

In *The Promise of Energy Medicine* Feinstein suggests that you can begin to "tap in your joy" using EFT. He explains that the first acupuncture point on the bladder meridian is at the third eye, and by tapping on your third eye when you are already feeling joy, you begin to repattern your nervous system around that feeling. He says that increasing your capacity for joy is a matter of opening natural channels that have become shut down. He suggests nurturing your radiant circuits which support joy and a positive attitude. You can learn to stimulate those points to activate endorphins and generate joy, at the same time you are flushing your body of negative energies. To learn tools to stimulate your radiant circuits read his book pages 249-265.

Byron Katie's book, *A Thousand Names for Joy*, is deeply spiritual work about how you can embrace everything through the eyes of love. I would highly recommend reading her book as you increase your peace and joy.

Louise Hay says, "If we could just make feeling better our goal, we could eliminate a lot of extra work." And in *The Path to Love* Deepak Chopra says, "For ecstasy overpowers all separation; ego gives way to pure flow of being."

The Bible says, "Rejoice always." Part of being in joy is being really present and not expecting anything other than what is. It's celebrating what is. William Blake captures this feeling beautifully:

He who binds himself a joy
Doth the winged life destroy
But he who kisses the joy as it flies
Lives in Eternity's sunrise.

There is an essential oil called "Joyful Moments" that reportedly opens your crown chakra and facilitates the relief of negative emotions. It contains orange, spruce, Frankincense, pine, myrrh, peppermint, fir and cinnamon. It might be worth a try. See www.livingfoodsinstitute.com under essential oils.

Unconditional Love

I found god in myself and I loved her, I loved her fiercely.

NTOZAKE SHANGE

Unconditional love is not something we learn about, discuss, or even strive for. In fact, I remember a fellow therapist once saying to me, "There is no unconditional love except between a parent and child, and if there was, I don't think it would be healthy." This is the logical ego mind talking, from the perspective of our physical world. It thinks that adult relationships should be reciprocal in order to be healthy and that we need to protect ourselves from being hurt emotionally and physically. Our Spirit self realizes that we are all One and that we can choose to act out of who we are, which is love, no matter what is happening around us. Most of us do not operate from that level of consciousness, but it is always available to us, both in a way that we treat ourselves and others.

Pema Chodron suggests using meditation as a tool to cultivate our capacity for unconditional love. She calls this practice tonglen. She says we should begin with a general feeling of goodwill and encourage it to expand. Perhaps you can think about something that makes you happy. She suggests we start with wishing ourselves happiness, then a friend, then a neutral person and then our enemies, and lastly we expand the feeling of loving kindness to all human beings. She says that Buddhist teachings say that over our lifetimes all beings have been our mothers. She suggested a mantra that made me smile, *"May this really annoying person enjoy happiness and the root of happiness. May this woman I resent awaken the bodhochitta."* That would make a great bumper sticker! She points out that difficult relationships are the most valuable practice.

I can imagine New Yorkers doing this kind of meditation on the subway. I guess broadcasting this mantra through the speakers would be unconstitutional, but it would be a great way to increase the collective vibration of unconditional love!

Journaling

For I will turn their mourning into joy, and I will comfort them, and make them rejoice from their sorrow.

JEREMIAH 31:13

Journaling was a great way for me to integrate and reflect on my cancer path and as a result, I'm going to suggest it for you. In fact, I'm going to take it one step further and when my energy is fully back, I'm going to create a Cancer Path Workbook so that you can journal your story as you go and create your own book. This is how effective I believe this process is.

When I was in graduate school I learned about Michael White's concept of Narrative Therapy and was particularly taken with it. White spoke about the importance of our stories in creating our identity descriptions. He developed Narrative therapy along with David Epstein as an attempt to help people separate themselves from their problem, while externalizing their values, beliefs, behaviors, and ideals. This in turn makes the person more aware of subplots, themes, roles and possibilities in their story.

In simple terms, becoming the heroine of my own cancer story allowed me to reflect on what I learned, what worked and wasn't working, where I still had to grow, the characters in my life and on my healing team and many other relevant issues. It allowed me to actively integrate a trauma and to take control over my life and story.

Anatole Broyard wrote *My Illness: And Other Writings on Illness & Dying*, saying, "My initial experience of illness was a series of disconnected shocks and my first instinct was to try and bring it under control by turning it into a narrative . . . Storytelling seems to be a natural reaction to illness . . . People bleed stories and I've become a blood bank of them."

Research shows that writing is therapeutic for patients with illness and cancer. One oncology study suggested that one 20-minute writing session may change how cancer patients think and feel about their diagnosis and have a positive impact on their quality of life.

In *Psychosomatic Medicine* a study reported that HIV patients who wrote about their worries for 30 minutes a day for four days straight experienced a drop in their viral load and a rise in infection-fighting t-cells.

In a small study at University of Kansas, researchers followed 60 women with early stage breast cancer who had just completed treatment. These women were divided into three writing groups. One group wrote their deepest thoughts about breast cancer. The second group focused on positive things that happened during their breast cancer experience and the third group only reported treatment facts. After three months, the first two groups who wrote about their feelings reported one-third fewer symptoms and medical appointments than the third group who only wrote about treatment facts.

In another study, researchers at the Lombardi Comprehensive cancer Center in Washington, DC revealed that expressive writing helped. They studied 71 adults with leukemia or lymphoma and had them journal while waiting for appointments. After writing, half of these patients said this exercise changed their thinking about their illness, and 35%,reported that writing changed how they felt about their illness.

Researchers at Dana-Farber Cancer Institute and Harvard Medical School in Boston found that expressive writing or journal therapy may boost mental and physical health in patients suffering from cancer.

A study at the University of Texas MD Anderson Cancer Center examined 42 patients with metastatic renal cell carcinoma (kidney cancer). In Phase II, clinical trial patients were randomly assigned to an expressive writing group or to a neutral writing group. In the Expressive writing group they wrote about cancer and in the Neutral writing group they wrote about health behaviors. Patients in the Expressive writing group reported less sleep disturbance, better sleep quality and duration, and less daytime dysfunction.

We don't necessarily need research to determine if something brings us therapeutic value. Personal experience is the greatest convincer. All you need is a pen and notebook to start a journal and there are no negative side effects. I wish there were more journaling or narrative therapy groups offered in hospitals , and I intend to start such a group in Manhattan, but you can always start one yourself with some cancer sisters. Others prefer to journal solo because it's a private space to be honest that no one can access. Try it and see if journaling is helpful to you. You will discover why and how.

Friends

There are two ways of spreading light: to be the candle or the mirror that reflects it.

EDITH WHARTON

Studies have shown that social support is important during illness. Researchers monitored students taking exams and discovered that the students who were most lonely had fewer t-cells. In another study of women with breast cancer, the women with the most social support had 30% more natural killer cells than those without connections. And in a study at University of California, researchers interviewed 5000 people in a big city and looked at how many friends they had and how many people cared about them. This included their community involvement. After 9 years, people who had few friends were twice as likely to have died as those with many friends.

Lastly, a study was performed with a caged monkey that was subjected to flashing bright lights and loud banging sounds, and then its cortisol hormone (which the body releases in response to stress and fear) level was measured. Cortisol represses the immune system. When another monkey was placed in the same cage, only half the cortisol was released. When 5 monkeys were in the cage, the lights and noises had no affect at all! By extension, the results indicate that supportive friends seem good for your immune system. According to Patricia Prijatel in *Surviving Triple Negative Cancer*, loneliness and lack of social outlets can lead to a surge in cortisol which allows tumors to grow through sugar and fat usage. In contrast, women with a strong social network were more likely to combat stress and disease.

Crisis is often a time to look at who is there for you. If you don't have people in your life who are capable of supporting you, look to build a new community. I have a friend who joined cancer groups and activities when she was diagnosed, and developed at least four new cancer friends that remained long after her cancer treatment. Be willing to reach out for help and to support others.

I made one good cancer friend named Jen, who I want to honor here. She is like a spiritual sister and made this path easier and more enjoyable. Since I lived far out of the city, had two kids and kept working throughout my treatment, I didn't bond much with other women who were walking through their cancer path. I consider it fate that Jen was both in my cancer yoga class and at the You can Thrive Foundation, when I attended. Not only are Jen and I around the same age, when we met we were both bald! We often would go out for tea together and hang out after class. Although she moved to Virginia and I stopped attending those classes, we remain in touch. Here she is:

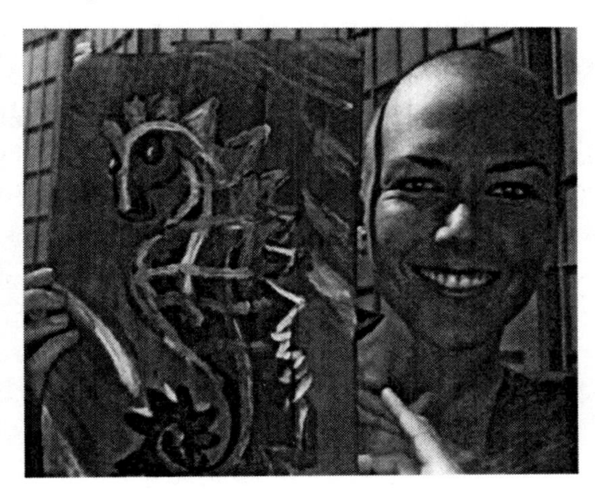

JEN WITH A HER SEAHORSE PAINTING

I asked Jen what she would like to share about her cancer path (which is hopefully almost over). She had Stage 3 breast cancer, HER-2 positive. She turned 36 right after her diagnosis & chose not to freeze her eggs because she was anxious to get started with treatment. She probably had been living with cancer for a few years at the time of diagnosis, and didn't want it to spread any more. She hoped that if it was God's plan, she might be able to still have a child one day, whether her own, adopted, or if she married someone with children.

So far Jen has had 12 weeks of Taxol (every week) then 12 weeks of FEC (every 3 weeks.) She also received Herceptin (which is an antibody) for an entire year, every 3 weeks. Then she had a full mastectomy and will still have a few minor surgeries to complete it. After surgery she had 25 days of radiation. She hopes to be all finished with her treatment by April 2013.

Jen said she's learned a lot from her path, the greatest of which was an increased spiritual connection. She worked with two spiritual healers, Katie Lamb and Eloise De Leon (whom she asked me to include in the Healers Appendix), and she felt they were enormously helpful. They gave her extremely reasonable rates and helped keep her energy high and strong. She used spiritual tools like meditation to support her journey. Every day she would imagine a cord going from her lower spine into the center of the earth with Mother Gaia holding her strong. Each day she would create a new cord connection. She'd also envision a huge rose, smell it, pick a color and thank it. With the rose healing, she would thank the rose for acting as a magnet for any negative feelings—hers, or those projected onto her from others. After it cleared her, the rose exploded like fireworks, transmuting the negativity into love, and sent it back to the original Source. Then she'd feel her aura around her and sense Source light and allow it to fill her up completely so that her whole body was glowing and her cells felt good.

She also paid more attention to her diet. She tried to eat lots of whole foods, especially vegetables, and she wants to juice more after her treatment. She also intends to buy organic foods and cook more, and make this an ongoing priority in her recovery. She allows herself a little sugar occasionally but tries to eat well 80% of the time.

She also learned how important nature was. It was her source of inspiration. She found answers to questions when she spent time alone in nature. She made offerings of many small trinkets, hanging them on trees in an area where she regularly hiked. She thanked nature and honored her breast and lymph nodes.

She also discovered the value of Western medicine, since her profession as an acupuncturist was far removed from Western style healing. Now she believes there is a place for everything and there should be more of a confluence of healing practices. She says that she asked her surgeon to say this to her during her mastectomy: "You will recover easily and quickly," and her surgeon agreed! I laughed when I heard this, thinking how we were similar and I had asked the medical staff to play an angel meditation on my iPhone during my port surgery.

Jen says that she has learned to focus on the positive and what's possible. For example, they removed 22 of her lymph nodes so right now she's not supposed to do yoga or rock climbing and many activities she did before. At first this really distressed her, but now she tells herself that there are so many new things she *can* do, and at least she's alive!

Jen looks forward to figuring out where she will live and where exactly she will be working when this treatment is all over. She's decided that she is ready for much healthier romantic relationships and is feeling ready to start dating again. She says she has become better at surrendering, reading the signs, and trusting and she is open to seeing where her path will take her next.

I'm so glad we met and her journey reminds me of how similar we all are, and also how unique.

Do you have a cancer sister? Why not reach out to one?

EXERCISE

Pick one or two events or places that you could meet other women going through this cancer path. It could be a cancer walk, a cancer yoga class, an organization, a cancer lecture, or a support group. Ask someone out to coffee and share what you've learned. It can be invaluable to find someone who really understands what you are going through.

Family

What can you do to promote world peace?
Go home and love your family.

Mother Teresa

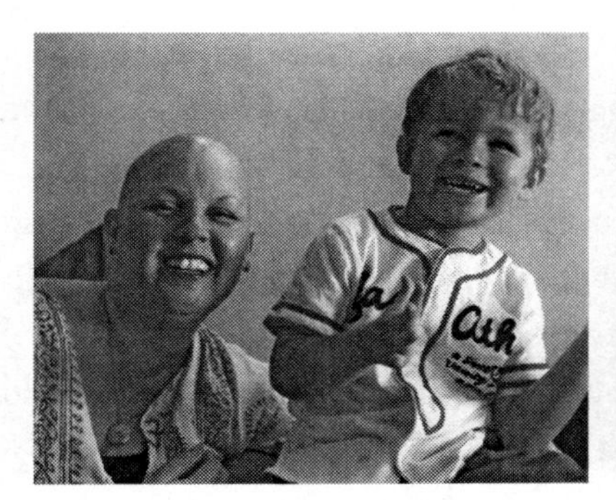

SON NOBLE & ME

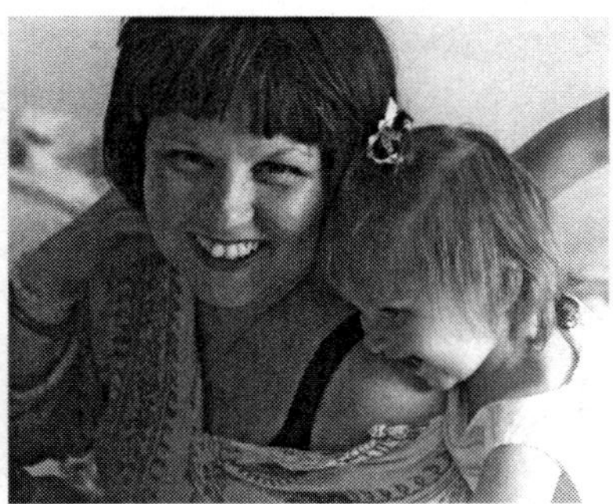

ME (WITH MY WIG) & DAUGHTER SERA

Often your family will be the people who are there for you day in and out, and you are lucky to have them. Hopefully they will offer you more support than agitation, but remember that they are going through stress and worry too and sometimes defenses emerge in fear.

There were times when I did not feel my husband or other family members understood or had empathy for what I was going through. Chris said that when I felt my family was being unsupportive that

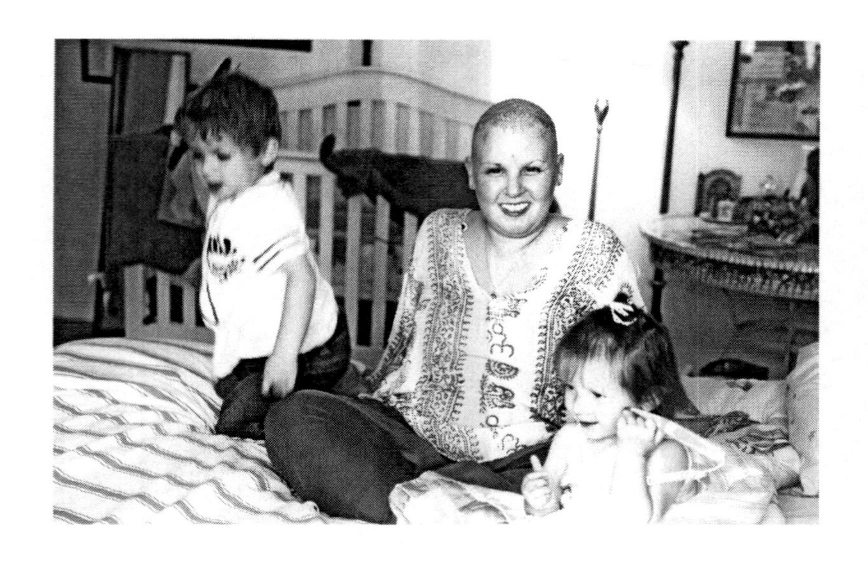

this loneliness was also an opportunity to develop depth and spiritual strength and resiliency in myself. When at times my husband and I weren't communicating well during this rough time, Chris explained that he was in a zone with me like in golf where he was "over par." For me, that meant I had to pray more and search more for love and answers within myself. Chris said that this theme would probably continue for a while as a means of promoting my spiritual growth. If I had a fantasy my husband would be hopelessly romantic and would make me green juice every day and ask me how I'm doing, this probably was not going to happen. He reminded me that many people are single, divorced, widowed or have an absentee spouse while they are going through a cancer path. He reminded me that my husband was good in many ways and better than the average guy. The more I let go of expectations and demands, the more likely he was to come through for me, although it felt to me like the more I asked of him, the less he would do. Chris said that I could have an intention or a vision about our dynamic, but he too was exhausted so I needed to let him make his own decision from his own motivation—and the more pressure I put on him, the more space he would need.

We can't force someone to give us compassion or care. Chris explained that my perceived lack of support wasn't personal, and if I were someone else my husband would be behaving the same way. Although some days I was under strain and wanted someone to hold me and tell me it was going to be okay, I couldn't compel that from my husband and I had to accept that. Instead I needed to find ways to give that love and comfort to myself.

One suggestion was to work on compassion and finding my own sources of joy, like a sunset or daisies. If I cultivated joy in myself that would sustain me. Contentment does not come from getting things—it comes from allowing things to be as they are. This sounded like a tall order some days, especially after chemo or radiation.

Ian picked me up twice a week when I was going through radiation so I did not have to deal with the 2-hour commute home after treatment and working all day. Then one day he was so frustrated from being stuck in traffic during rush hour that he took it out on me, yelling that from then on I had to take the train and he was done picking me up! I was so mad and tired. I didn't have the energy to fight. I asked for Divine Guidance before going to sleep that night and woke up from a dream that said, "You can have Heaven or Hell. Choose."

I took that to mean that I could fight or find a peaceful solution. We were all under a lot of stress so I just decided to take a car service home the next three weeks and then I'd reassess my schedule and hopefully my energy would be back. So, consider choosing your battles during treatment

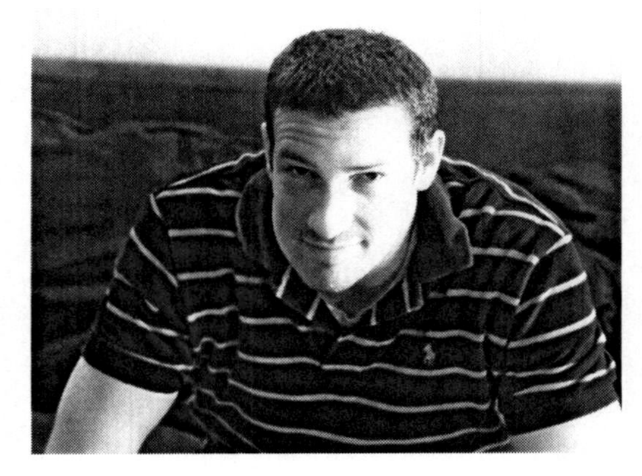

MY HUSBAND IAN

To My Beautiful Wife,

I know I may not express it very much but I am very proud of you - getting through this battle with a high head and Great Spirit - It is very inspiring to see you move forward with your dreams despite the obstacles. I also feel how much you love me and our family. I am blessed for that. I love you very much,

Your loving husband and Pillow

because everyone is stressed and on overload. Instead of looking for love out there, try and be love. Try and give it to yourself. You deserve it.

Having told the above stories, I should say that my husband does give me a lot love and care. I shared these snapshots of my intimate relationship because during stressful times you will have expectations of your spouse, boyfriend, and family members, and you may also forget that they too are going through stress, hopelessness, and exhaustion. Sometimes they will deny this to themselves and to you. Truth be told, my handsome, sweet husband has put up with a lot of challenges and we've gotten through them all together. I know I'm very lucky and I love him very much. And it helps to remember all that when he pisses me off and we're both sensitive and sleep-deprived.

In general, I believe in most moments that the purpose of this cancer path is a calling in my Spirit for sustenance. There are more people going through this experience on their own, who are feeling alone and unsupported. They will also have those surprise moments of sweetness from others and they will have disappointments. In the end, the biggest gift may be to learn how to rely on yourself and to realize how strong you truly are.

Although my husband didn't say much as I went through all this, he surprised me with this card that meant a lot.

Thanks, honey.

Cancer is new and scary, and friends, family, and caretakers may express their fears and feelings differently than you would. Do you best to notice how they do show that they care. Acknowledge that love and let it in.

How Feelings May Affect Your Body

One of Candace Pert's books, *Your Body is Your Subconscious Mind*, explains why the subconscious mind is the source of psychosomatic illness. Her breakthrough discovery was that neuropeptides are in every part of the body so all our cells are intelligent entities. She showed that emotions are produced directly at the cellular level as "molecules of emotion." These emotions trigger the entire body into an altered state of consciousness where emotional states switch our physiology. This important discovery reminded me that our emotions do affect our physical health and this is something our doctors should ask about.

In the hospital they put up this chart of emotions (see below) on the wall but no one mentioned it otherwise. Doctor visits were very scientific and it seemed like how patients were feeling was largely insignificant. Only physical symptoms were usually discussed in terms of pain, not the emotional pain of all the changes and possible pending death.

Why is it that you are asked to report your level of physical pain but not your emotional pain?

My radiologist oncologist met with patients weekly and handed out questionnaires about their emotional state where they could appraise their emotional pain on a Likert Scale. On the bottom of the paper it said this would be forwarded to a nurse or social worker if the ratings

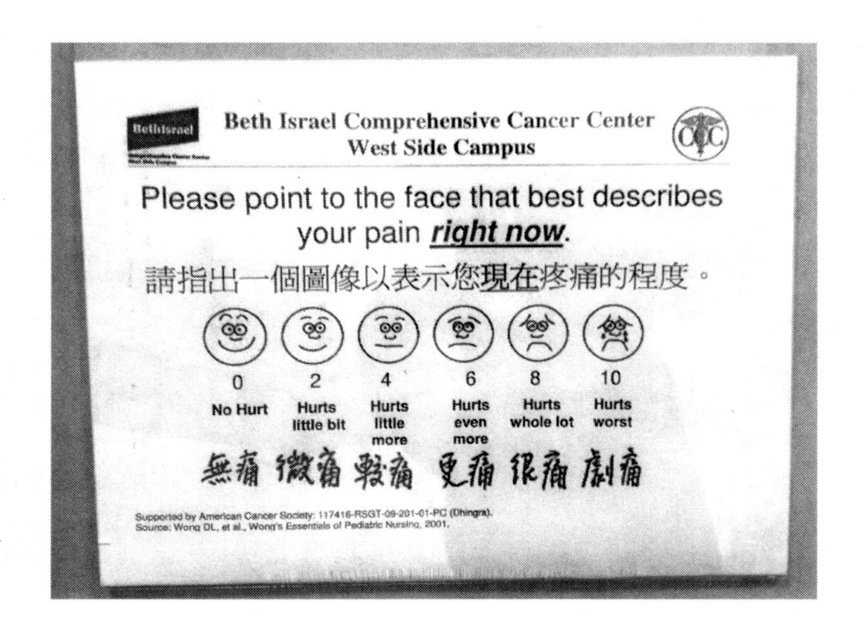

were above a 3. It impressed me that he went this extra step to consider the whole individual that he was healing because I had not encountered this with any other doctors. I suggest that addressing the patient's emotional pain is something that all medical students should be trained in. I also think that there should be a social worker on the team assigned to each case who would at least meet with every patient once to assess them. Cancer patients may need assistance in processing feelings and loss and should at least get a referal to an affordable great counselor. Since no one offered me that option at the hospital, I decided to offer counseling and cancer coaching to patients and to try to explain the importance of this option to hospitals.

Dealing with Hospitalizations

I had the fast growing conviction that a hospital is no place for someone who is seriously ill.

NORMAN COUSINS

Going to the hospital can also be hard. Many people think hospitals are scary places—and indeed, if you are in a hospital, it's because you or someone you love is unwell. Hospitals are associated with crisis, illness, surgery, medicine and death. For my cancer treatments I was in the hospital for the lumpectomy, every other Friday for chemo, and every day for 6 weeks for radiation. But at least then you know it's for routine treatment. A few of my cancer friends unexpectedly spent the whole weekend there due to organ problems from the chemotherapy and high fever.

As I write this section, we just got back from a whole day at Maimonides Hospital for my 1 1/2 year old daughter Sera. As I mentioned, she has Alagille syndrome, a genetic disorder that can affect the heart, liver, and kidneys. She has peripheral narrowing of the arteries and they have to give her EKGs every few months, but she is too small so she doesn't sit still. So today they scheduled us for a sedated sonogram and EKG, and they put her to sleep. I was nervous because there's a chance she could stop breathing, but it all went well.

It's hard to be in the hospital all day with a toddler. Anyway, this sweet child life specialist named Jon Luongo brought her stickers and bubbles today. He was playing with wands with her while she got her needle and went under and I was really touched that someone (besides us) was addressing her Spirit and her emotional needs. Here's a picture of her brightening up from that experience.

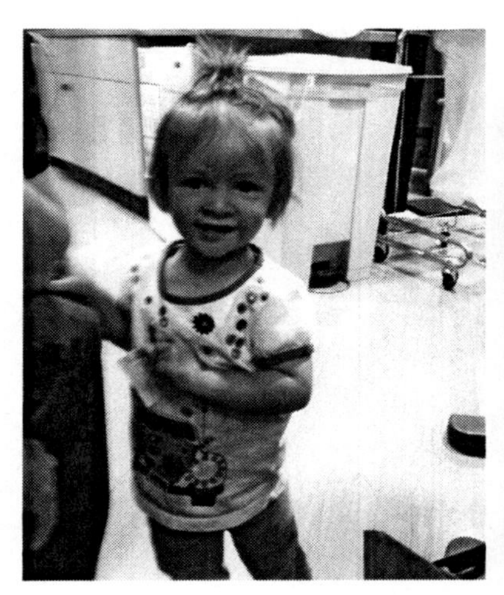

SMILING SERA HOLDING THE STICKER SHE WAS GIVEN

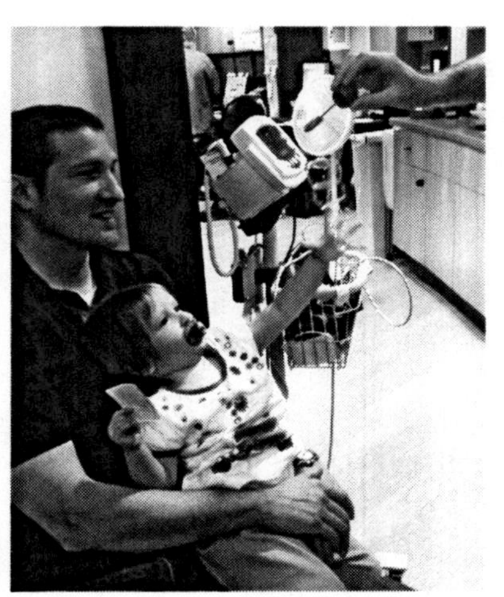

SERA REACHING OUT FOR BUBBLES IN THE HOSPITAL

I had the song that she was named after, "Que Sera, Sera" on my iPhone and she loved it. She could sing most of the words even though she was only 19 months old. Music was a good mood elevator for all of us.

It would also be helpful if hospitals had a designated person for adults in the hospital too. Maybe we've outgrown bubbles but it would be great to have someone walk around to cancer patients to tell jokes, hand out magazines or flowers, or just talk. I truly feel that addressing each person's Spirit is as important as addressing their body in the healing process. Doctors deal with many life and death crises daily, but for the average person being in a hospital is emotionally draining and frightening, and most people aren't accustomed to it.

Having said this, there is usually no one like that during your hospital stays so if you think you might be there overnight, think about how to raise your own spirits, improve your environment, and distract yourself. Now with the iPad you can watch Netflicks (movies), or listen to music or comedians. You can bring books, magazines or your journal and even look at pictures of your loved ones. The possibilities are endless so see what works best for you.

SECTION IV

Spirit

All the way to heaven is heaven.

St. Catherine of Sienna

All of us have a soul. It is the immortal part of us that's connected to the Divine. It is our proof that we are all One, from the same family. In a poll, 90% of respondents said that they believe they have a soul but few had experienced it.

I think this will change and we will be brought into circumstances that encourage us to engage our spirit more—circumstances like cancer. We currently come from a culture that is fast-paced, materialistic, and very earthbound. If people can't see their soul then they don't know what to do with it. They've come to trust their eyes and taste more than their intuition. Perhaps this is because they were never shown how to connect with Spirit.

In my experience, science is experienced as the antithesis of "the unknown," or spirituality, and there is no room in science to make meaning of one's illness in medicine without material proof. This paradigm is shifting however. The issue was brought to light in the film starring Meg Ryan, *City of Angels*, where a doctor has a spiritually transformative experience and realizes that healing and life and death choices often happen in partnership with God. Many doctors have had near-death experiences, completely changed their framework and written books about their experiences, and I have referenced those books here. In addition, new programs in spirituality and medicine and narrative medicine have sprung up in California, Missouri, Minnesota, New York and other places.

Research is demonstrating the importance of spirituality in a patient's life and healing. A recent study by Phelps et al. reported that 78% of patients with advanced cancer relied upon their religion to help them cope with their illness. McCord et al. administered a questionnaire to patients in waiting rooms and 87% wanted doctors to inquire about their spiritual beliefs. Balboni et al. reported that 72% of advanced cancer patients reported unmet spiritual needs by the medical system.

Dr. Christina Puchalski is the Director of the George Washington Institute for Spirituality and Health in Washington, DC. She has pioneered clinical strategies to address the spiritual concerns common in patients facing illness. She invented a tool called the FICA Spiritual History Tool to help doctors and residents systematically assess a patient's spiritual history. An evaluation of her tool found that most patients rated belief or faith as very important in their lives.

Hopefully, you will have an enlightened doctor ready to help you along your spiritual path but assuming you don't, in this section we will continue to explore how connecting with our Spirit will help in life and along on your cancer path. I think Spirit was the single most compelling element for me to heal. We will discuss how prayer, meditation, signs, dreams, nature and more can connect you at a soul level. We will explore how having a spiritual context can help you learn life lessons and remain in a state of love instead of fear or pain. Deepak Chopra writes, "If you can bring your attention to the level of soul, struggle ceases." He also says, "Healing is a broad term; being connected to both whole and holy. It can be defined spiritually as a return to the state of unity."

Spirit can also help you understand how to use your God-given gifts and reveal how God can use you to spread love in the world. According to Donna Eden, the soul is the source of most subtle energies of our being. She says that it infuses our body with life and our brain with consciousness. She says that the deeper we enter the lives of our personal soul, the more we will identify with a universal intelligent Spirit and the better our bodies will fare. So, there may be even more connections between body, mind, emotions and spirit than we yet realize or understand.

Similarly, Dr. Hawkins says that general growth in spiritual development brings about health and can do so rapidly if we are willing to let go of limiting beliefs. He explains that paradoxically, spiritual work may bring repressed patterns into manifestation. This is characteristic of mystics who frequently go through periods of illness. He explains that saints descend to the bottom of the scale prior to achieving a higher awareness. He also states, "Spiritual endeavor and intention change brain function and physiology and establish a specific area for spiritual information in the right-brain prefrontal cortex and the etheric (energy) brain."

Connecting with a higher energy can bring peace to your overall physical vibration. As John Steinbeck once wrote, "A sad soul can kill you quicker than a germ."

I hope this section will enliven your Spiritual life in new and lasting ways. I will cover some spiritual tools that helped me on my cancer path that might also be a point of inspiration for you.

Your Soul's Mission

This little light of mine. I'm gonna let it shine . . .
let it shine, let it shine, let it shine!

HARRY DIXON LOES

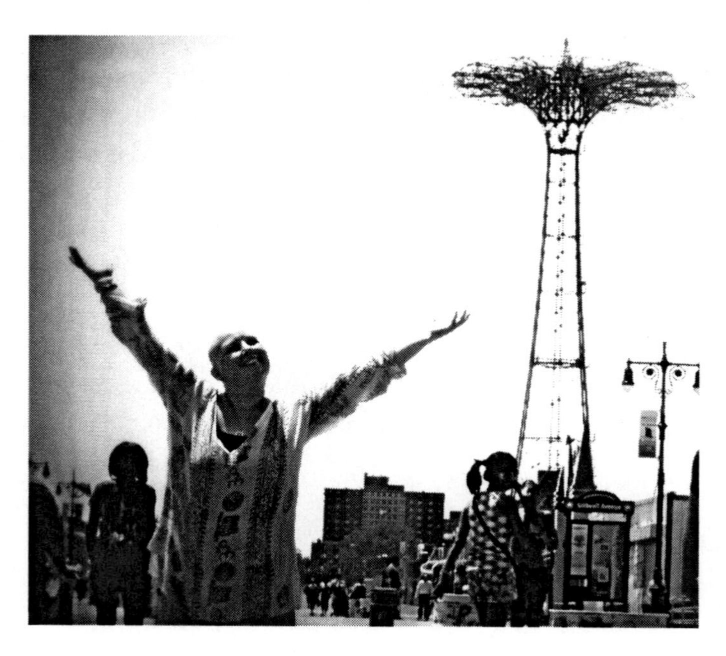

PARACHUTE JUMP PUBLISHING
"BOOKS THAT INSPIRE YOU TO LOVE MORE."
WWW.PARACHUTEJUMPPUBLISHING.COM

In *Gift from the Sea*, Anne Morrow Lindberg wrote, "One must lose one's life to find it," and I have found this to be true. Knowing and fulfilling your soul's mission might be something you examine once you are faced with your mortality. It was an immediate topic of consideration for me. Cancer was the zen stick to help me get crystal clear on why I am here and to take action on it.

The first thing I noticed is that my Spirit stepped right in when I was diagnosed with breast cancer. It's almost as though there was an instant reassurance that I was not alone. When you are faced with your mortality you immediately ask the big questions like, "Did I do what I came here to do? How was my life?" At least, I did.

Fortunately, I felt pretty happy and relaxed about the answer. I loved and was loved and I had accomplished most of what I'd wanted to create. I wanted to marry my soul mate. I wanted to have a boy and a girl and buy an apartment on the beach. I wanted to do work I loved and publish a book. Check, check, check, check. But then I heard my Higher Self say, "Yes, you've lived the life you set out to live but you have 22 books to write still. This is your legacy too." Of course I thought, *22 books! Are you serious?* It sounded exhausting yet I knew it was true. My family complained when I wrote one book because it took lots of time and didn't bring in much income. Nonetheless, the soul doesn't care about material returns like that.

I wondered if this was my soul or my ego talking. I knew that my ego pushed me to accomplish things but that my driven nature had also pushed me down the cancer road away from self-care and balance it seemed.

I continued to finish the book I was writing, *When Mars Women Date*, while I underwent my lumpectomy and at the beginning of chemotherapy. One thing that changed was since I'd been given a soul's directive, I had no time to waste. I didn't know what the cancer had planned. Before, I was going to send sample chapters to agents and try to find a publisher, which seemed largely out of my control. So I decided I would take it in my own hands and self-publish. I'd start my own publishing company and just put my books out there myself! I knew that they'd reach the right people and I would do my part. This realization and choice felt like a relief, even though I had so much work ahead of me. I had no idea how to publish a book (much less 22) but I knew I'd figure it out. And, if this was my divine purpose, I'd be shown the way.

So, although most people around me seemed negative about my seemingly wacky idea, I forged ahead with my plan. My sister, who visited with her boyfriend Albert when I was first diagnosed, has a Ph.D in English literature and she tried to discourage me from writing. By her standards I wasn't very good, plus she knew I had no time and wouldn't make much money from my books. Instead she encouraged me to eat better foods, join a cancer support group, listen to angel tapes she'd brought me, and as you know by now, it was she who insisted I call Chris, the angel guy in California. I agreed, happy to be taken under my big sister's wing at the time.

So instead of getting a therapist or support group, I called Chris, or Christopher Dilts from www.askanangel.org. During our first session I told him about this feeling I had that I was supposed to write 22 books. He gave me validation, assuring me that it was my soul's purpose. He told me that doing this would bring me healing energy and I should tell myself that "my mission is stronger than my cancer." He said that having a purpose larger than myself would compel me forward through the cancer path. I completely agreed.

He told me that higher powers wanted me to do the book that I was writing (and future books) would also come through me. My book, *When Mars Women Date*, was mostly done at that point but he proceeded to tell me why it was important, what it was about, and how it would cause a shift in our mass consciousness. This was exactly my vision for that book and for our society so with that confirmation he had my attention.

He told me that my creative energy was far stronger than any disease, and I had gifts from God to share that were more powerful than any internal or external resistance. This is what I already knew in my heart. I decided to keep writing throughout my cancer experience, with the intention that this cancer path could help me heal myself and inspire others to do the same.

I tell you all this because for me, focusing on a project greater than myself gave me a positive focus beyond the cancer and a drive to complete things, which was a powerful context. It may help you too to write or to think of a meaningful way to contribute to the world. Next, I will be creating a workbook called *Your Cancer Path Workbook* that will help you document and reflect on your experience as you go through it. This could be the raw material for a book of your own.

Anyway, Chris said I needed a place of proof that Spirit could help me by undergoing the cancer treatment. I needed to journey up the spiritual mountain to know the Divine Mother in all of her forms and I needed this cancer challenge to go that deep and to pause long enough to renew my Spiritual connection. He said this journey was necessary for me to call on support from higher levels. If everything remained cushy I might not have gone there and my soul knew this. To my soul the most important thing was evolution and sharing my gifts. This (cancer) experience did not take place because I was bad or was being punished. (This might be something you were thinking and that you need to hear too!)

Breast cancer is now 4 times the national average and rates are 50 times higher than 50 years ago due to our environment and stressful lives. Hundreds of millions would be climbing this same cancer mountain and it is always easier to take on a challenge with company.

Of course, you don't have to feel that if you do not have a soul's mission that you are lost, but perhaps getting cancer will incite you to look at this for yourself. For some people, a soul's purpose is their creative work, career, family , charity, or doing something they love. I have a friend who had always wanted a house of her own. She worked for her sister as a secretary to pay the bills and then she'd spend all her time fixing up a cute, dilapidated house she bought, filling it with her love and creativity.

To find your purpose, think about your gifts and what you would do for free, just because you love it! Ask people who know you, or better yet, meditate and ask your Higher Self. Moving toward your purpose will focus you and will bring you passionate energy. You can also get a reading with someone like Christopher to find out more about what your purpose is.

Author Sonia Choquette says that your soul's mission is in every cell in your body. Our job is to reactivate what's lying dormant in our consciousness and activate our Higher self's commitment to your true nature. I truly believe that your passion activates your vitality and will to live.

When my sister visited me she brought me a birthday care package. In it were two Sonia Choquette books and some angel cards and statues for my altar. I started reading one of the books and it felt like a perfect synchronicity. Sonia prefaced her book by saying that her guides told her to divide her book into 22 sections because the number 22 is a sacred number that reflects how the physical world is manifested. She added that the Hebrew alphabet has 22 letters and there are 22 archetypes in the major arcana of the tarot deck. I later read that Dr. David Hawkins said that there were 22 sages on this planet who calibrate at level 700 or higher on his Map of Consciousness. All this got my attention since it just so happened that I was writing 22 books as my legacy and I don't know why.

I recommend Choquette's book, *Soul Lesson & Soul Purpose*, which can guide you in 22 things you can do to live from your Higher Self.

In my next session with Chris he said that my cancer was like a Zen stick from my soul, telling me to change a lot of habits. My soul was guiding me to do things that support me better emotionally, physically, mentally and financially. This would put me on a narrow path with my diet and my presence would increase and I'd be of much greater service to people. I needed to keep my vibration high and to stay on purpose. He said that my book would be actualized without much effort and I should just keep asking my angels for help.

He told me that this was breast cancer because the breast is the most feminine part of the body, and it provides milk to feed others. The root chakra represents the Divine Mother's milk of love and forgiveness, so healing that chakra would nourish me with things like juicing, alone time, chi gong, etcetera. He said I would no longer need to use brute will to accomplish things with my mind. I would start to use a power greater than me and shift into my heart and Spirit more so that I'd have help and allow things to flow. He said that cancer would make me more open, softer, and more willing to listen. And I think in some ways it has.

As I continued to read Sonia Choquette's book, she explained that our personal vibration rises as we master our soul lessons. She says that your soul chooses your circumstances, including your family, body and where you are born, in order to serve your evolution. She says that trauma snaps you into the present and says, "Wake up!" She tells readers to say to their Higher Self, "Higher Self, use my mind, heart and body to serve humanity and create my fullest potential."

For me, cancer lessened my fears of judgment and perfectionism concerning my writing. I just wanted to get my message out.

I wanted to write from my Spirit or essence and not be pushed to exhaustion by my ego, hounding me to accomplish. I responded to something I read in *Emergence* by Barbara Marx Hubbard who wrote, "The workaholic aspect of my local self subsided. For the first time in a long time, I felt at peace . . . always placing my attention on my life's purpose rather than upon the evolution of my self . . . my work had been taken over by attachment and compulsion . . . there was a shift in focus from doing to being . . . allowing it to come forth unimpeded by anxiety, self-criticism, as a flow of creativity . . . the key to practice at this stage is to continue to put essence first, not second." While this was sound advice and a great marker on the path of evolving your soul's mission, I noticed I'd go back and forth between ego and essence. But something new was definitely breaking through. I was standing in my truth and that light would shine through, whether people liked it or not.

My husband put up a shelf near my altar at home where I could put my books as I published them. Seeing it every day was a great source of inspiration, to remind me of my legacy.

Here it is so far:

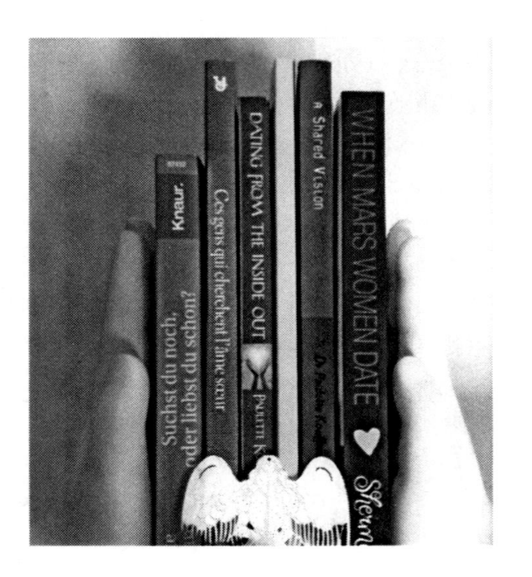

There are 4 books here (plus a couple versions in different languages). This cancer book you are reading and 2 other cancer books will make 7 books in all (once they come out), plus one children's book. Then there are just 15 books left to go in my Legacy Project (see www.parachutejumppublishing for more information)!

So, getting crystal clear about my soul's mission really helped me move forward.

If this interests you than I'd suggest meditating or walking alone in nature. Ask your Higher self your purpose here. Think about your gifts and how you can share them in the world. Then journal about the messages that come to you. It may seem simple or modest but that's okay. Carolyn Myss says that Spirit most often seems humble but that's how you know you are onto something major. Just be willing to take the first step!

Solitude

Certain springs are tapped only when we are alone. The artist knows he must be alone to create; the writer, to work out his thoughts; the musician to compose; the saint to pray. But women need solitude in order to find again the true essence of themselves: that firm strand which will be the indispensable center of a whole web of human relationships.

ANNE MORROW LINDBERG

For me it's been very important to spend some time alone, to connect with my Higher Self and be creative. I've gotten grief from some extended family members who feel as a mother I should always be with my kids. Still, spending time hearing the voice of my soul helps me heal, refuel, achieve my life mission and ultimately be a better wife and mother.

Everyone needs time alone and it is usually in stillness and solitude that we can hear our Higher Self. There was the image of the magus or healer in one of my old tarot decks and he/she is going into a cave. One has the feeling that you have to go within and affect your internal environment before you can create miraculous changes out there.

One of my favorite books, *Gift from the Sea*, was written by Anne Morrow Lindberg who would spend some time at the beach in solitude, away from her husband and five children. One senses what an important spiritual pilgrimage this was for her in her prose, and as a result, she touched the lives of many. As a result of her experience and writings hopefully many more women and people are carving out this time for their soul, creativity, and healing.

No doubt it can be challenging in our busy world of technology and responsibility, yet it is possible and necessary, as one can usually hear the voice of their soul best in silence and solitude.

Walking this cancer path I found that the person I relied most upon was me. No one else could get the chemotherapy or radiation. No one else could completely understand how I was feeling. I went inward for answers and comfort and avoided many outings with friends. For me it was enough to work, see my husband and kids, write, go to the hospital and see friends occasionally. I did not attend a lot of groups, nor did I desire much outside stimulation. For me the path was inwards and perhaps cancer set the stage for people to understand "no" more; at least, some people. And to those who thought I should be doing more caretaking during this experience, I simply said, "Oh well." For me this alone time was precious and sacred. It was part of the process of calling back my soul to heal.

This doesn't mean the same thing must apply to you. Perhaps your sacred path takes you outwards and reconnects you to others and to your community. This can be just as profound.

You may find that for you healing means letting yourself be supported by others. Just make sure that you are not running from yourself or from being alone. This is your chance to befriend yourself too and to find a wise, strong, ever loving inner core that will always be there for you. Spending time in solitude opens this door so I hope you'll explore walking through it.

Your Higher Self

The eternal is internal.

Paulette Kouffman Sherman

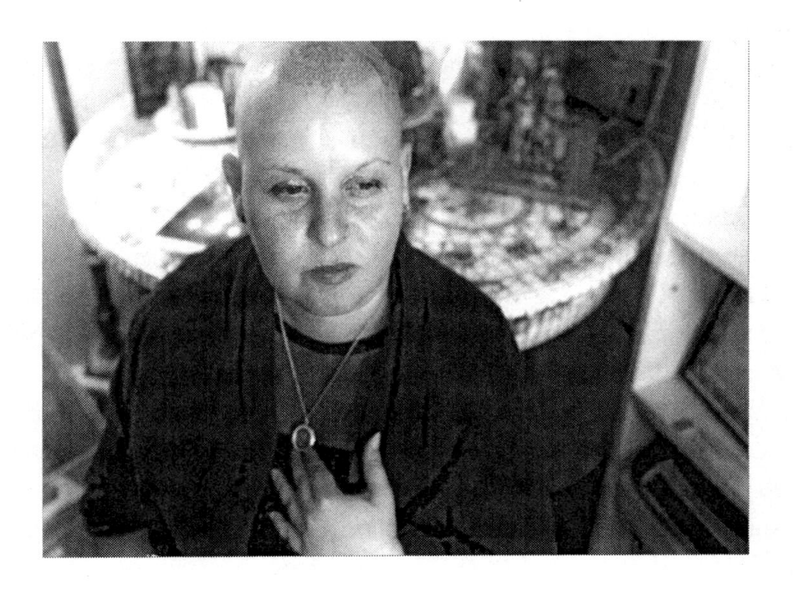

Your Higher self is your guidance system in this lifetime, your divine guidance. It wants your Spirit to accomplish your mission on earth. It lives eternally and rests in your soul, giving you wisdom about your mission and gifts. It has a Unity consciousness, Divine Mind and sense of oneness. An appropriate quote here is, "The Kingdom of Heaven is within."

When I walk on the beach, sometimes I try to get messages from my Higher Self or I will ask it questions. I think it's easiest to hear your Higher Self when your environment is quiet and you are relatively still and empty. Today I listened to see whether I received any wisdom. I heard, "What you resist, persists. You need good self-care to be as successful a teacher as you wish to be, otherwise you won't be able to hold so many responsibilities and demands. It will just be even harder than, if it's not a set habit. Also, life is meant to be fun and enjoyable. When you drive yourself too hard you are separate from your body and Spirit. Everything is One. It's Love. You feel that you can't balance it all but life is not a competition or a race. Remind your ego that in the Life Review in Heaven, massive accomplishments don't matter. What matters is the love you share and what you learn here."

I find that listening to my inner voice is very helpful and I'm starting to do it more. It's important that we embody our own wisdom so we don't always have to source it "out there." As Deepak Chopra says, "Wisdom isn't something you learn, it's something you become." In *The Path to Love* he says, "Spirit responds to your vision of it, and the higher your vision, the more you will evolve." I also love the quote by Schiller, "What the inner voice says will not disappoint the hoping soul."

Oprah Winfrey once said, "It isn't until you come to a spiritual understanding of who you are—not necessarily a religious feeling, but deep down, the spirit within—that you can begin to take control."

Your Higher Self is your proof that you are One with the Beloved and Spirit is you, not just something out there. Barbara Marx describes this as "Get[ting] to the is-ness of yourself as the Beloved." In *Dying to Be Me* Anita Moorjani writes, "Heaven is a state not a place . . . I became the Source."

Make your Higher Self your best friend and compass, and your whole life will unfold in beauty.

Levels of Consciousness

The pure love of one soul can offset the hatred of millions.

Mahatma Gandhi

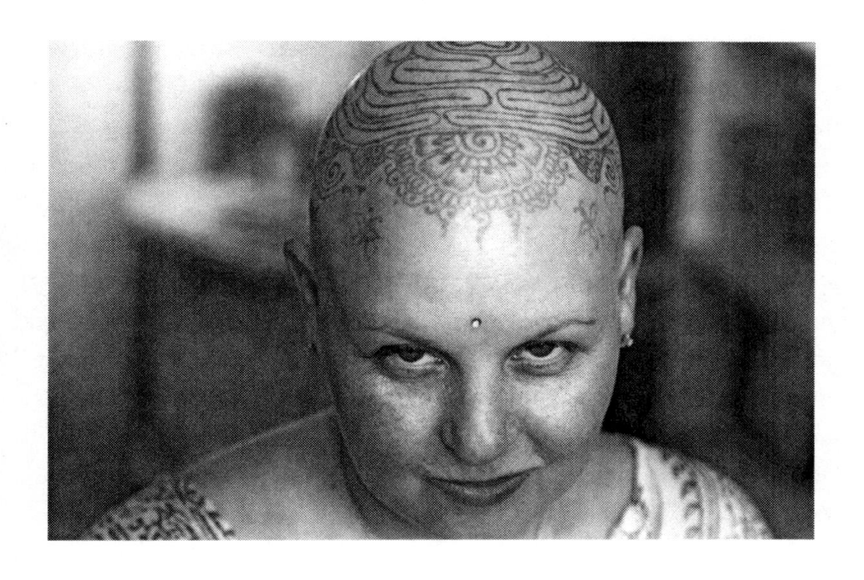

One of my favorite books is *Transcending the Levels of Consciousness*, by Dr. David Hawkins. I like that he self-published a large body of his work and has continued to make such a difference, even now, after he has passed away. About a year ago, I had Googled "levels of consciousness" and discovered this book, never having heard of Dr. Hawkins. In it, Hawkins describes how over a two-year period he cured himself of a number of serious illnesses. I liked his book so much that I found his website and learned that he was 88 years old and was giving his last lecture soon. It was a Higher Self moment and I clearly knew that I had to go to Sedona, AZ, to see him speak. I did not know how this might happen, but I told my husband and he miraculously agreed to go with me for the weekend. Grandma babysat our two kids, we flew there after work, rented a car, stayed at a motel, heard him lecture all day and then saw Sedona in 3 hours before flying home. I thank my husband for humoring me and honoring my inner voice. I did not get to personally meet Dr. Hawkins but it was nice to see him in action on stage. This man was on purpose!

Dr. Hawkins devised a "Map of Consciousness" with calibrated levels of consciousness on a logarithmic scale from 1-1000. He says that a third of the world lives at the bottom of the map in states of fear, grief, and apathy, that 78% of humanity is below 200 level of consciousness, and that 49% of people in America are below 200. According to Hawkins, 200 is the level we can discern truth, and that to a large degree health is an expression of our level of consciousness. Under a consciousness of 200 these energy fields potentiate illness and pull adversity into our energy field. There is adrenaline and survival response released from energy fields under 200. They potentiate left-brain dominance, fight-or-flight mode, alarm, a lowering of killer cells and the immune system, increase disease and serotonin. He says these lower energy fields are like clouds covering the sun.

The energy fields above 200 support healing. From calibration levels of 200 up, there is a release of endorphins and feelings of pleasure and happiness. These energy fields are right-brain dominant and engender peace, endorphins, increased immune system functioning, increased killer cells and healing. He says that only .4% of the world population vibrates at the level of unconditional love. Hawkins writes that moving toward the top of the Map of Consciousness reflects not what one does, but what one is.

Only 1 in 10,000,000 people attain the level of peace at calibration 600, according to Hawkins. The good news is that the enlightenment of one person can counterbalance the negativity of 70,000,000 people who calibrate below 200. And even for those who reach level 500 (love) they will counterbalance 750,000 individuals who calibrate below 200. So, according to Hawkins, raising our personal level of consciousness is raising the collective consciousness as well. What we do for ourselves effects others. He says, "The collective consciousness is like the level of the sea; as the level goes up, it raises all the ships on the sea."

Hawkins explains that parts of your life will calibrate at higher levels of consciousness and parts will calibrate at lower levels. We can bring awareness to our shadow areas, and ultimately it's the average of all these levels that determines our overall consciousness.

Illness often follows the beliefs we hold in the mind. All illnesses are physical, mental, and spiritual, and the highest recoveries arise from addressing all levels. Hawkins says, "If we look at the basic physics of the energies involved, we can see why fear, which calibrates at 100, is overpowered by love at 500."

He believes all people are born under optimal circumstances for spiritual evolution and as we evolve spiritually we're tested to see if we pick ego or divinity. Saying that catastrophe can be a good way to learn, he quotes the Zen teaching, "Heaven and hell are only one tenth of an inch apart." This rings true to me these days!

Dr. David Hawkins Map of Consciousness is a great visual representation of levels of consciousness and how we ebb and flow in our states of consciousness. It helps us to notice where we are at any moment and to move up into the higher ranges. This practice can help you shift from ego to essence, increasing your spiritual power.

EXERCISE FOR RAISING YOUR CONSCIOUSNESS

Here is a good context for you to try when you are scared or angry. Close your eyes and say to your Higher Self:

"Help me to see love, safety, peace, and acceptance in this situation."

You can also ask your Higher Self, *"What would LOVE say?"*

Then journal about the messages you receive and apply them to your situation.

If You're Doubting or Limiting God's Power

In the fulfillment of the will of God lies the power of the human soul.

Bensei Douno

A friend recommended that I read Harold Kushner's book, *When Bad Things Happen to Good People.* Kushner's son died at 14 years old from a rare disease, and this caused him to deeply question why bad things happen to good people and to assess God's role in such events. He concluded that God does not prevent or cause tragedies but is there to comfort us and give us strength once things do happen. He says that some human tragedies we bring upon ourselves (like the Holocaust) while others are just bad luck.

My views on God differs from his but many people find his book helpful because it points out that bad things do *not* happen to us because we are bad and God is punishing us. He says that an attitude like that creates guilt, causes people to hate God and themselves, and makes them turn away from religion. He points out that life isn't fair and there may *not* be a reason that bad things do happen. He feels that prayer and religion can rally community support, which is helpful during tragedy.

His limited view on God's role in our life's tragic events may or may not appeal to you. I put it here as an opposing context to karma or the idea that we go through challenging experiences to learn about ourselves and raise our consciousness. As you know by now, I tend towards the latter.

Each of us is different, though. I realize that some of you may believe in a limited God, some of you may believe in an unlimited God, and some of you may not believe in God at all. Hopefully whatever your stance you can find something that illuminates your spiritual journey in this book and allows you to feel connected to something larger.

Keeping the Faith

There are two ways to live: you can live as if nothing is a miracle; you can live as if everything is a miracle.

ALBERT EINSTEIN

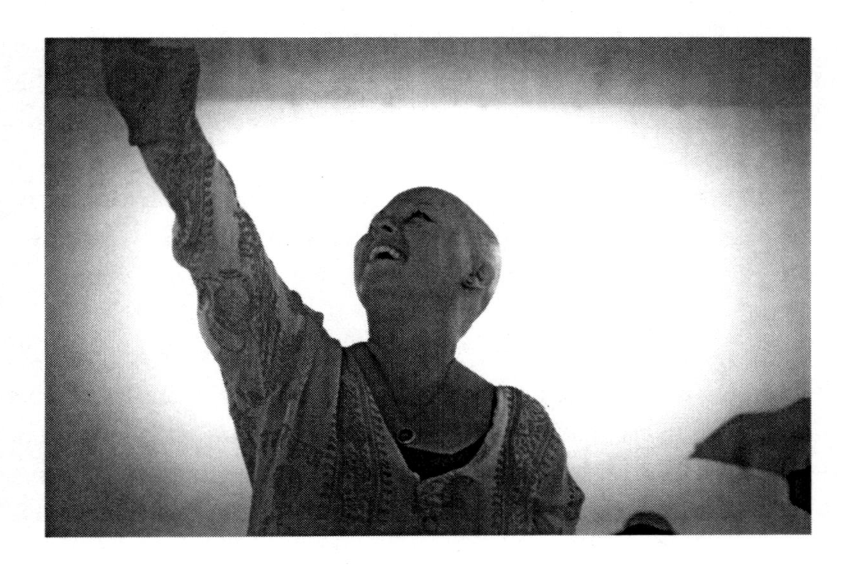

Maintaining my connection with spirit was one of the most helpful factors in maintaining my sense of peace and purpose after being diagnosed with cancer. Even though I consider myself spiritual rather than religious, I can appreciate biblical stories that convey how important faith can be to get us through challenging times. They remind us to look within to ourselves as a Spirit rather than to judge our worth and safety from external conditions.

Into this new love, die
your way begins
on the other side
become the sky

Rumi

One such story is the biblical tale of Job. Job's belief in God was severely tested. All of Job's possessions were destroyed: 500 yoke of oxen and 500 donkeys carried off; 7000 sheep burned, 3000 camels stolen, and the house of the firstborn destroyed, killing all of his offspring. Still, Job did not curse God. He shaved his head, tore his clothes, and said, "Naked I came out of my mother's womb, and naked shall I return: Lord has given, and Lord has taken away; blessed be the name of Lord." The story ends with Job restored to health, with a new family, and with twice as much livestock. He doubled his riches and lived 140 more years.

In *Energy Anatomy* Carolyn Myss suggests that, like Jesus, we will all undergo some sort of test or betrayal and will feel victimized. This helps us to see how much we are plugged into human order instead of divine order. Our faith is tested so we can learn to trust more and then our consciousness rises. We learn to love more unconditionally in this process because we plug our Spirit back into Source.

Having faith often means trusting and surrendering to what happens, knowing that God has a larger plan for us. In *To Heaven and Back: A Doctor's Extraordinary Account of Her Death, Heaven, Angels and Life Again*, author Mary Neal tells the story of drowning and visiting heaven before returning to earth. She recounts, "It has taken me many years to learn that when everything seems difficult and feels as though you are swimming upstream, it is usually because you are not following the direction of God's will. When you are doing God's will everything seems to happen without much effort or many obstacles . . . If you transform your faith into trust, you can face any challenge with a grateful and joyful heart."

I also found it interesting that even research shows that what you believe (whether it's real or not) has an effect on the healing outcome. *The Placebo Effect* shows that just believing in a drug's healing effects can help overcome a physical illness in up to 50% of cases. In *The Promise of Energy Psychology* Feinstein reports that people who believed that they were prone to heart disease were nearly four times more likely to die from it than people with the same risk factors who did not hold that belief. Feinstein says that holding a belief that something negative will happen has an even stronger impact than having a placebo belief.

Clearly the belief in an unconditionally loving presence who will support you through challenging times could be protective and helpful. For me, God and the angels could be there when friends and family weren't, and during the times when I wasn't being supportive to myself. It is an adjunct, not a substitute for these other things. But if you believe in the Divine, it can help you embody a higher vibration of love at any time.

In addition to having faith outside of yourself, having faith in God can help you become more reliable. Swami Sri Yukteswar said: "Forget the past. The vanished lives of all men are dark with many shames. Human conduct is ever unreliable until anchored in the Divine. Everything in future will improve if you are making a spiritual effort now."

The Spiritual Meaning of Illness

He who has a why to live for can bear almost any how.

NIETZSCHE

The spiritual meaning of illness became a focus on my cancer path. My husband and many doctors thought that getting cancer is just genetics or dumb luck. I'm not psychic and I cannot tell you that there's definitely a spiritual root to all illness but my gut says that things usually happen for a reason and it's our opportunity to learn why, at least for our own satisfaction.

The psychologist in me also felt that if you just treat the symptoms and not the root cause that whatever it is you're dealing with could return. I won't say that this applies for you and I don't say it to scare you either. It's merely another point of consideration on your path. Your oncologist will probably just want to kill the cancer but you can wonder about any spiritual message it might be bringing you. As Christopher Dilts once said to me, you can say to your cancer, "Hello my friend. What have you brought for me today?" And then listen.

I also wondered whether this cancer experience might have been part of the contract I signed on for when I was incarnated, in order to learn from cancer and help others through it. Author Sonia Choquette says that we pick certain experiences in this earth school to learn from. I remember when I was in graduate school in Pennsylvania I used to love going to the Borders bookstore there, and would often attend the author events. One day I randomly sat in on a book signing for *The Eternal Journey*, a book about near death experiences. It was written by two researchers who interviewed many people who had physically died before returning to their bodies. One woman had fibromyalgia and she had been bitter about it most of her life. When she died she flashed to a scene where she was in a sort of classroom with an angel. The angel told her that on earth you learn fastest through suffering, and one quick way to progress was to have fibromyalgia. He asked if there were any takers and this woman remembered raising her hand. Then she went back into her body and resuscitated. After that she lived her life with fibromyalgia by teaching people about it, with a renewed sense of purpose. I love that story and have always remembered it.

But there are other perspectives on suffering. I once visited my high school friend Rachel's house when she had a sort of guru named Harry visiting. He asked me what I thought life on earth was about. As a result of the story I just mentioned, I said, "I think we are here to learn from our suffering." And he replied, "As long as you think that, there will always be suffering." This was quite a profound statement and completely reframed my context. Unfortunately we didn't have a chance to continue the conversation and I never saw him again, but his response stays with me. Now I think a re-contextualization could be that we have trials so we can learn to love more and create our world. We may experience challenges but we can accept them or suffer. In her book, *A Thousand Names For Joy*, Byron Katie says something similar to what Harry said: "Your suffering can't show me the way. Suffering can only teach suffering." What do you think?

As a child of a Holocaust survivor, I remember reading Viktor Frankl's iconic book, *Man's Search for Meaning*. He wrote about how even in a situation where there were seemingly no choices (in a concentration camp), he could choose his attitude and use his imagination. He shaped his own psychological life despite incredibly painful circumstances. This is a powerful book and I recommend reading it.

Right before my lumpectomy surgery I rented a video from Netflix called *Fierce Grace* with Ram Dass that I would also recommend. This spiritual teacher was paralyzed from a stroke and had to relearn most things, including talking, which was an integral part of his teaching ability. He discusses how this hit his ego but it eventually took him deeper spiritually and allowed him to have greater compassion and understanding for people suffering similar losses.

Also, even if we have the same illness, there may be a different soul lesson for each of us. When I spoke to Christopher about the spiritual meaning of cancer for me, he offered a few things. He told me that I had a brilliant mental body but that I had been in my mind creating things for a long time. He used a funny metaphor saying, 'Your mind is like an arrogant executive in the penthouse suite looking down at those other chakras in your body saying, "Who has time for you? Look at my brilliant self. Look at my view of Central park! Isn't it beautiful?" He continued, "But we need those lower relationships to make it all work. Look at what's happening now on Occupy Wall street in the financial district!" His analogy made me laugh but it rang true. We all need to work together in this world and this takes a philosophy of wholeness.

I rationalized that my family needed me to make money so that we could afford to buy a house and send two kids to college. I had cut myself off from nature, my body, and even my Spirit to some degree as a result.

Chris also said that cancer would teach me to deeply attend to the needs of my body and to be more aware of energy, while learning to merge my mind and my heart. He cited research showing that the energy field of the heart was 3000 times more powerful than the mind and that it would create an even greater attractor field around my books. He said I had the consciousness and sensitivity for this work and now the cancer was creating the willingness, which would require me to make many changes in habits on my part. He warned me it wouldn't be easy.

He quoted Yogananda who said, "The mind is a great slave and a terrible master." He explained that my mind wanted me to learn everything and to grow more brilliant but what I really needed was to go deeper not to *do* more. He said I had enough knowledge and now I just had to practice simple things that would not take a lot of my time like 3-part yoga breath and my root/crown/heart meditation and invoking my angelic maitrix on a daily basis. He explained that breathing was important because most spiritual masters stress that "quality of breath equals quality of mind." I understood that knowledge needed to be embodied and this could best be done through good habits and practice.

I could see how cancer had provided a context for me to be open to slowing down and to balance these areas, change my habits, and do some forgiveness work for myself and others. I also think it has made me much closer to the energy of the Divine and to my spiritual purpose. These are all great gifts that cancer has brought me. Sometimes I think that I understand why I may have chosen this experience on a spiritual level before incarnating, exhausting and painful as this path has sometimes been.

THE SPIRITUAL MEANING OF YOUR ILLNESS EXERCISE

I'd like you to take a moment to journal about any spiritual lessons you've learned from having cancer. And, if you believe that we choose our major life experiences before we incarnate, why might you have chosen to experience cancer in this lifetime? This exercise may help you be response-able for this path, instead of being pulled along as an unwilling victim of your circumstance.

If you can embrace your spiritual lessons and gifts you can share them with others. This process can be transformative and life-giving.

Karma: I Wouldn't Hurt a Fly?

The highest development of the human being is someone who has come to the complete end of suffering himself or herself, and therefore will never create suffering for others.

Sharon Salzberg

The Buddhist concept of *karma*, according to Daniel Goleman, is described as "the process of cause and effect in which motives and actions produced by physical and mental effects for the person engaged in the actions, as well as for the recipient of the actions." Others say through our actions we create our own rewards and punishments. Karma is also a process by which we affect everything else. Ted Andrews describes karma as, "situations chosen on a soul level that provide a continuing spiral of growth."

The Dalai Lama says this about karma: "Decisions should be made on the basis of what is beneficial and what is harmful. It is consequences that determine whether an action is right or wrong. Any action that leads to a harmful consequence can be judged wrong, and an action that leads to beneficial consequences can be considered a right action."

In her book, *Angels are Talking*, psychic Michelle Whitedove says that our every thought, word and deed has a reaction or consequence that comes back to us. She says that if we hurt or judge someone, we will eventually volunteer to experience being the victim of that set of circumstances. Whitedove believes that we draw up a blueprint that includes our karmic debts from past lives and that our soul stores our past deeds like a celestial debit card so we know what needs to be repaid—once a lesson is learned, that debt is repaid.

Michael Mirdad (*Healing the Heart and Soul*) says that when we evolve spiritually we experience "instant karma" rather than the long-term payment plan of reincarnation. He says that everyone accepts at least one cross or issue to bear in order to remain dense enough to stay embodied. He says we can begin to feel grateful to those who have hurt us and forced us to go within and embark on Soul-Level healing. He says, "You can learn to see the 'cross you bear' as a focal point for healing through forgiveness—not only to release yourself but also to release everyone on the planet with the same issue."

You've heard the expression, "I wouldn't hurt a fly," and know that we often associate this phrase with Tibetan monks, who live according to the concept of right action, which includes not harming any living being. Well, I'm no monk, but I do try to live by this rule as well—but I do have a fly story. Some time ago, I was up early in the morning (during treatment) and I was taking a shower. There was a big noisy fly buzzing around me and it scared me (at the time I did not think it was a fly). I thought of swatting it but it also crossed my mind that it isn't good karma to kill anything. So, (I'm embarrassed to say) I took a wet wash cloth and put it over the fly, thinking this wouldn't kill it but would allow me to finish my 10 minute shower in peace. I fully intended to let it out afterwards. My children suddenly started calling me and making a ruckus so I quickly finished my shower and my husband went right in after me. Without speaking about it, he must have picked up my washcloth and let the same loud fly out. He probably had no qualms about killing a fly and proceeded to swat at it with a towel. Somehow the fly got underneath the frame of a picture of the beach that we have hanging in our bathroom and died there! See below:

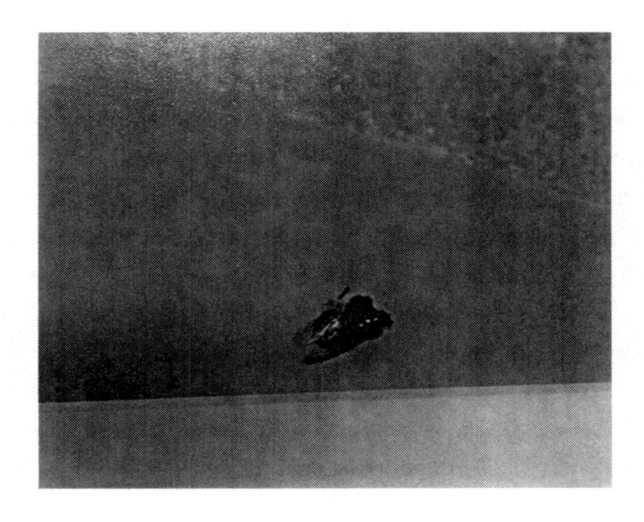

FRAMED FLY WHO FLEW IN OUT OF FEAR AND DIED AS A RESULT

It is a rather gruesome ongoing reminder of karma. Maybe that's why I haven't moved it out of the frame. Recently I was in the shower and a mosquito came in and was flying all around me. I said aloud, "I don't like mosquitoes," but I somehow refrained from swatting it. And so goes spiritual progress, I guess.

Most of us aren't monks but we move through our days trying to be good people . . . so why do we see a fly as unimportant? We make arbitrary distinctions between life and death. Consider the chicken and burger we eat versus the cat or dog we nurture and protect. Perhaps we are all just trying to juggle and get through the day and we feel we can't afford too much consciousness or we'll go crazy. I'm just admitting my own tendency to slip into fear or laziness, and silly as it is, the framed fly reminds me that it's not just extended family, coworkers and homeless people we need to strive to be kind to, it's every living thing. And of course, we may never achieve perfection.

In the New Testament, Jesus's disciples asked about a blind man and Jesus replied, "Neither this man nor his parents sinned, but this happened so that the works of God might be displayed in him." (John 9:2-3). So perhaps we really need to look at karma not as punishment but as a loving opportunity for growth.

In terms of our karma, we usually have one or two core issues in a lifetime. Mine was practicing my self-care and underneath that issue may be that I did not feel worthy. Chris said I should make sure I am not trying to be an author in order to be loved by others. He said we can't look for love outside ourselves because people are fickle. He said I can have my motivation to help others without expecting an outcome. My job is to show up, be receptive, and do my best.

My friend Brad, Director of "Intuitive Energy," says that sometimes something looks one way from our physical body but our spirit knows it's karma and is something meant to serve our spiritual evolution. He gave an example of someone wanting to understand the legal system as a Spiritual being, so they reincarnated as a criminal in this lifetime to learn about it from that vantage point. His point was that things we view as "bad" are still opportunities for our spirit to learn in the larger picture.

There is also Group Karma which is a lesson that large groups of souls inflicts upon another group of people. This lesson usually revolves around prejudice: racial, religious, economic or intellectual, etcetera. The dominant group that perpetrates the injustice must repay the karmic debt. Author and psychic Michelle Whitestone says the Holocaust is an example of how group karma affects mass consciousness, as it has long effected Germans, Jews, and all of us. She also mentions what she calls "A Victim Soul," which is a person who has chosen to soak up a large amount of karma for humanity in this lifetime (this could be people who perished in the Holocaust, or Jesus Christ, for example).

Oneness

Is it really so that the one I love is everywhere?

Rumi

I think a lot of what we do, think, and feel derives from our context: whether we view ourselves as part of a larger, whole system or whether we think of the world in terms of competition—as in, "survival of the fittest." Our ego often navigates the world as though we are in a race to compete and win but our Spirit knows our lessons and love are eternal and we are all One.

We all start life with a oneness consciousness and then slowly lose it as we create our personal ego identity. My daughter Sera is almost 2 and she is very smart. She knows everyone's names. I asked her her name and she smiled coyly, saying "Kim." The next time I asked her name, she replied, "toy." She knew she was stringing me along, and she knew that I knew what she was up to. She acts like she is equally in love with the entire universe, even strangers. We go to a restaurant and she smiles and offers literally everyone licks of her lollipop! When did we lose this sense of our oneness?

If you want to try a new practice, go through your day and say, "I am One with that" to yourself. Notice how it makes you feel and respond differently to other people and circumstances.

Peace

Until there's peace in you, there is no peace in the world,
because you are the world, you are the earth.

Byron Katie

Byron Katie discusses peace as it relates to cancer in her book, *A Thousand Names for Joy*. She says, "How do you know that you need cancer? You've got it. . . . Do you think your body is going to heal most efficiently when you're tense and fearful and fighting cancer as an enemy? Or when you're loving what is and realizing all the ways in which your life is actually better because you have cancer, and from that calm center doing everything you can to heal? There's nothing more life-giving than inner peace."

Penny Peirce asks in her book, *Frequency*, "What have you allowed to be more important than your inner peace?" I think it's a great idea to sit a moment and really ponder this. Is it a fight with a friend, your weight, your money situation, or your cancer? Is anything worth sacrificing peace in this moment? Your answer to this question is a choice and it has long-reaching implications for yourself and others.

Sacred Places & Rituals

In fact the word 'spiritual' is a combination of the words 'spirit' and 'ritual.' So, it could be said that our spiritual path is a journey filled with rituals and initiations.

MICHAEL MIRDAD

When my sister and her boyfriend Albert visited after my diagnosis, they suggested visiting a cemetery where the revered Rabbi Menachem Schnearson was buried in Cambria Heights, Queens. He was buried at a place called *Ohel*, which means the resting place of a righteous person. It is said that you could put a letter on his grave and your wish would come true. It sounded like a fun excursion and I was touched that my sister wanted us to wish for my recovery and good health, so we went. She happened to mention our pending trip to my son's preschool teacher, Sara, who happens to be married to a rabbi, so they both came with us to the cemetery and showed us what to do and told us some of the history. We learned about the Rabbi Shnearson, we all wrote a letter, ripped it up and made a wish, after lighting a candle. My husband and children came as well, so there were 6 of us doing this ritual together. It was a sacred night. If you would like to visit the grave site, you can find more information at www.ohelchabad.org. The grave site is open 24 hours a day, six days a week. There are even directions on the website for how you can send in a letter and have them place it on the grave site for you, if you live far away. This was an extraordinarily compassionate, wise man who reportedly performed many blessings and miracles, so asking him for a wish couldn't hurt. It was also a sacred night because of the ritual and being in the presence of loved ones who were holding the space, with uplifting intentions for me and my health. I felt very blessed.

You may choose a different kind of ritual to bless your cancer path. In the book, *Rituals of Healing*, a healing ritual is described as any ritual whose purpose is to make whole. In Navajo culture, severe sickness is treated by long "sings" where loved ones gather for days.

Other than the above ritual at a sacred site, I was thinking about what rituals I've performed during this process. I got a henna crown or a henna tattoo on my bald head, with the design of a labyrinth with a heart center. To me this represented my Cancer Path that would lead me deeper into my heart and healing. I also walked regularly on the beach to the Parachute Jump and said my prayers there.

I also started a daily practice of meditating and involving the Divine Angelic Maitrix, plus I would usually fall asleep to my angel tapes. Sometimes on Friday nights my son Noble would remind me to light the Shabbat candles, to bring more light to the world.

I've heard of women who have mikvehs (Jewish ritual baths) after chemotherapy, who take sacred site vacations, or climb a mountain.

What rituals bring you Divine energy and comfort?

Songs

If music be the food of love, play on.

Shakespeare

Music can be very therapeutic. Rhythm acts as a natural tranquilizer and it is said that chakras in our body vibrate to certain tones. Music expresses emotions, makes people feel less alone, and can connect you with courage, hope, love, and strong ideals in the midst of trauma. In my graduate school dissertation, "Playing Among the Dead," I researched how Holocaust survivors employed creative strategies to survive psychologically during trauma. Many of them sang and used music to keep their Spirit strong and to continue to feel human. Brown (1989) explains that music animates emotions below conscious feeling and can dramatically effect one's physiology. The roots of auditory nerves are more widely distributed and have more connections than any other nerve in the body. Sustained chords can lower blood pressure and crisp repeated chords raise it. Harmonious rhythms can be sedatives or stimulants, depending on the tempo.

Sometimes when I woke up in the morning before going to my cancer treatment I'd sing songs that inspired me to create a great tone for my day. There's a song by Olivia Newton-John called "Grace and Gratitude" that put me into a state of appreciation. Her lyrics are, *"I thank you for life. I thank you for everything. I stand here, in grace and gratitude and I thank you."* You can choose your own song and sing yourself into the mood it evokes. Sing it in your bed, in the shower, on the subway, in your car, and while on your way to work or to the hospital.

The other day when I was walking from my radiation appointment to work, I caught myself singing a song that my sweet son always dances and sings to, and it brought me such happiness. I sang, "If you've got troubles and you need a helping hand, come with me I will be your friend. I will be your friend, I will be your friend. If you've got troubles and you need a helping hand, come with me I will be your friend!" I could picture his smiling face and the music had such a catchy melody that it carried me all the way across town in no time.

Sometimes I would sing my son the Joan Baez song, "Heaven Help Us All" when he was going to sleep. To me it's a good reminder of why we are here. When I wanted comfort I also loved the song, "I'm Here to Mother You," by Sinead O'Conner.

What songs move you? Make a healing tape of songs that speak to your Spirit.

Music does transport you, reminds you of what's important, connects you to your heart and eases pain, and it has long been used as a way to communicate with the psyche and spirit.

Some inspiring songs for breast cancer survivors are Melissa Ethridge's song, "I Run for Life," and Martina McBride's song, "I'm Gonna Love You Through It." I also love Olivia Newton-John's CDs, "Gaia," "Grace & Gratitude," and "Stronger Than Before." She was a breast cancer survivor too.

Music can be a direct route to your physiology, emotions and soul. It will sometimes be the medicine that can get you out of bed in the morning or make you feel that life is worth living. Emily Dickinson put it best when she wrote, *"Hope is the thing with feathers that perches in the soul and sings the tune without the words and never stops at all!"*

MUSICAL EXERCISE

Take some time to make some mixed tapes. One can be songs that comfort of inspire you. You can make one tape with healing songs, including music of dolphin sounds, and you can even make a tape of sad songs that you can cry to if you need a day to feel sad. This will be your own music therapy that you can use as a tool whenever you need it. I still like mixed tapes but if you are more advanced you can use mp3s from iTunes and put the playlists on your phone and computer too.

Visualization and Collage

As much of heaven is visible as we have eyes to see.

Ralph Waldo Emerson

I've always been a maker of Vision Boards. I feel that visualizing something and laying it out makes it more likely to happen. Vision boards concretize your vision on paper. With visualization, you practice seeing what you want in your mind.

Research on visualization is mixed. Six studies in 2005 suggested that guided imagery may be helpful in managing stress, anxiety, and depression for people with cancer. One study showed that visualization improved the mood of people having treatment for breast cancer. A clinical trial in 1999 involving women with early stage breast cancer found that guided imagery helped ease anxiety related to radiation, breast surgery, and the recurrence of cancer.

A review in 2005 looked at guided imagery as part of cancer treatment. It found that guided imagery might provide psychological support and comfort. There was no evidence it helped with physical symptoms such as sickness and vomiting but results were positive enough to justify more research.

A review of 46 studies in 1999 suggested that imagery may reduce pain, and some of the side effects of chemotherapy. One study suggested that imagery can reduce anticipatory nausea and vomiting from chemotherapy. Imagery is considered one of the more useful psychological measures to reduce some side effects of chemotherapy. Some studies suggest imagery affects the immune system.

In a study of imagery and mental rehearsal on basketball performance, volunteers at Ohio State University were divided into 3 groups. One group practiced shooting free throws every day for 30 days. The second group did the same thing, but only in their mind. The third group had no instructions. After thirty days all three groups came back to shoot free throws. The third group who did not practice at all had no improvement. The ones who had practiced real basketful improved 24 percent and the ones who had practiced only in their minds improved 23 percent! This finding amazed me and confirmed for me my intuitive sense about the value of using visualizing and creating vision boards to shape outcomes!

In the book, *Getting Well Again*, Carl Simonton adapted visualization techniques learned in Silva Mind Control to treat cancer and mobilize the body's defenses. The Simontons describe a six-week program for cancer patients to change negative attitudes, with relaxation and visualization sessions three times a day. The patient identifies stresses and examines the benefits of illness. They recommend physical exercise three times a week and finding sources of inner guidance and goal setting.

Jeanne Achterberg and Frank Lawlis developed a scale for rating the intensity of imagery for descriptions and drawings of cancer cells and white blood cells. Nearly three hundred patients were interviewed and evaluated in three studies. The imagery session often involved picturing cancer cells being destroyed in treatment and a story that ends with the patient healthy and free of cancer. They could visualize themselves reaching their goals and fulfilling their life's purpose. In the cases where the patients died or their condition deteriorated, the evaluation of their images predicted the course of their disease with 100% accuracy. For those who entered remission, their image scores predicted improvement with 93% accuracy. This is an astonishingly high level of predictive accuracy, and it is exciting to see that mental images can reflect the internal physical processes of cancer patients.

Dr. Bernie Siegel's books, *Peace, Love and Healing, and Love, Medicine and Miracles*, combines psychological and visualization techniques. His groups with patients examine dreams, drawing, and imagery, and he teaches his patients how diseases like cancer and AIDS can be an opportunity to find the meaning, love, and joy in life. He tries to understand the emotional experience as the disease developed, and the function of the illness in a patient's life. Then he has the patient draw a picture. The picture is usually a self-portrait or a representation of the patient through symbols. He then works with the patient's self-images and appreciation for life, to produce a stronger sense of self and develop a positive purpose for living.

In the classic book *Creative Visualization* by Shakti Gawain, she gives clear directions about how to begin a daily practice of visualization. Visualization, she says, is the technique of using your imagination to create what you want in your life. She suggests that you count down from ten to one after fully relaxing and start to imagine something you'd like, such as being radiantly healthy. You can add affirmations like, "I am healthy and feel strong and energetic." She suggests doing this for 15 minutes in the morning and evening, after getting into a relaxed state. She reports that her mother dissolved her gallstones without surgery using visualization, but she recommends that people try this as a supplement to their regular treatments.

In another study, after being instructed in how to use visualization to inhibit the breakdown of red blood cells in a test-tube located in a different room, experimental subjects achieved statistically significant results in their efforts to slow the rate of cell deterioration.

In the book *Rituals of Healing*, the authors explain that imagery acts as a bridge between the various functions of the body mind, which responds to images "as if" events that are imagined are actually happening in the outer world. Visualizing a picture activates the visual cortex and imaging sounds stimulates the auditory cortex.

How can you use visualization to help you through treatment and healing? Louise Hay recommends visualizing cool clear water washing away your diseased cells or creating a vision where love dissolves all the cancer cells. She also says to tell yourself when you are in surgery, "Every hand is a healing hand."

My spiritual mentor, Christopher Dilts said, "God is in radiation too. The Divine is not separate. Picture the Divine releasing cancer cells and bringing them back to Source. Breathe in deeply during treatment and receive the Divine Mother's love. Feel deeply loved and cherished and valued."

Gloria Steinem once said, "Without leaps of imagination, or dreaming, we lose the excitement of possibilities. Dreaming, after all, is a form of planning."

Doreen Virtue teaches progression, which is a visualization that takes you forward in linear time to see your future life and goals so you can learn what you need to manifest those goals.

Personally, I like a method called *Silva Mind Control*. Jose Silva knew that the ideal mind circuit was the one with the least resistance that would make the greatest use of the brain's electrical energy. He found that at lower frequencies the brain stored and received more information. So, he used a combination of relaxed concentration and mental visualization to prove that we could function with awareness at alpha and theta brain frequencies. He did 39 experiments to prove that he trained children in ESP. The most inexpensive way to learn his method of visualization is to buy his small book (listed in my appendix) but the organization also runs workshops and sells DVDs. They teach you to easily enter an alpha state of consciousness and to picture what you want on a mental screen. In the alpha state you are processing the good health images more deeply than if you were telling yourself this in a beta (alert wakeful) state.

Creating a vision board or a collage makes your inner vision concrete. I have always loved collages and I do them for various goals and phases in my life. You can also do collages about painful experiences like cancer in order to integrate the experience. Artwork can be a way to achieve distance from what's happening physically and provides a safe way to express traumatic images whereby the artist maintains a sense of personal control. It also provides a transitional space where the artist can disown the affects and memories of a trauma and can serve as a testament and legacy, something concrete to leave behind. It also serves as a bridge from their internal experience to the broader community.

For these reasons and more, it can be very helpful to draw or make a cancer collage. Maybe it can even be a treasure map leading you from being bald and in treatment to having flowing long hair and accomplishing your dreams while being vibrantly healthy. Research shows that the unconscious responds to imagery and this could be an inspiring graphic representation of your path.

Cancer can be an isolating and disorienting diagnosis until you can integrate it and connect with Source. Employing your creativity can be very helpful in this process. It requires going deep within and then finding your way back into the world. Goethe captured this when he said, *"Art is at once our greatest refuge from the world and our surest connection to it."*

COLLAGE EXERCISE

Create a collage of your cancer path. Collect some pictures of you now and then cut out pictures from magazines of places you'd like to travel and what you'd like to do. Show yourself getting through the cancer treatment and manifesting all these things in your life, including radiant health and wholesome eating. Then hang it somewhere you will see it regularly so it will inspire you. Here is mine:

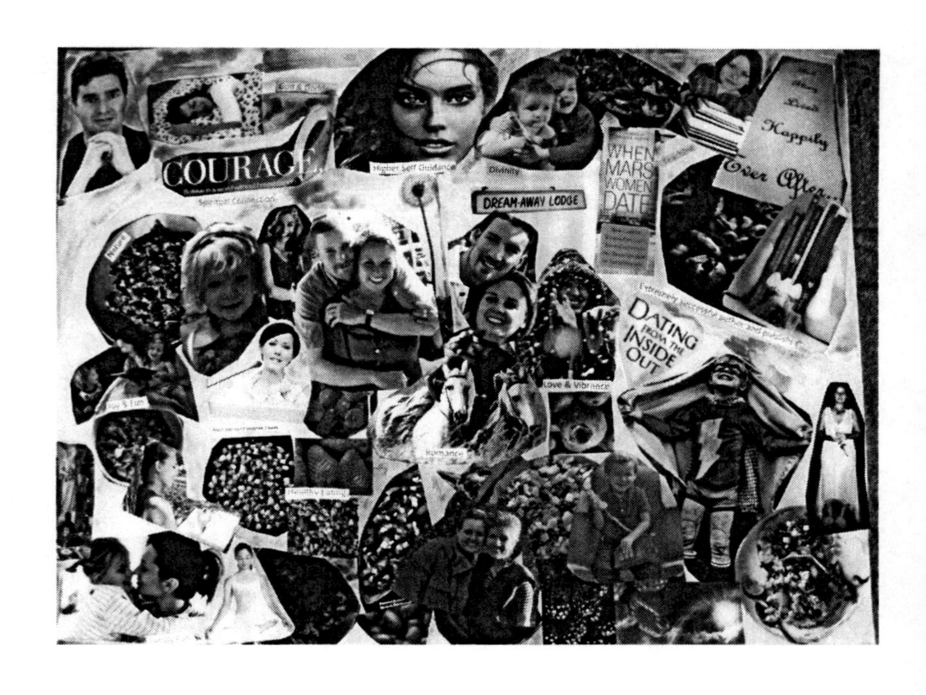
COURAGE
Higher Self Guidance
Divinity
DREAM-AWAY LODGE
WHEN MARS WOMEN DATE
Happily
Ever After...
Nature
DATING FROM THE INSIDE OUT
Love & Vibrance
Joy & Fun
Romance
Healthy Eating

Vibration & Frequency

Stop acting so small.
You are the universe in ecstatic motion.

RUMI

A great book on vibration and frequency is Penny Pierce's book, Frequency. She talks about how everything is vibrating energy and we each have our own personal frequency that she calls our "home frequency." We have 4 types of brain waves: Beta, Alpha, Theta and Delta and they correlate with our levels of awareness. In fact, she says that the slowest brain wave states (Theta and Delta) correlate with higher frequencies and expanded awareness. These are the brain states achieved through meditation, which is why it is considered an imperative component of any spiritual path. She says that as our ego begins to dissolve, we can achieve a more expanded soul awareness. Whatever you materialize embodies your vibration in some way, and as a result, illnesses or injuries correspond with inner blueprints that are based on negative emotions that relate to the afflicted body part.

This made me think about what was in my personal vibration that might draw in cancer. Louise Hay says the breast is nurturance and that breast cancer has to do with self-care. I think that has been something I have been working on more diligently since getting diagnosed.

Yet, simultaneously, I feel like this path has connected me much more deeply to my soul's vibration and has raised my home frequency as a result.

In his book, *The Healer's Manual*, author Ted Andrews addresses vibrational remedies including gems, colors, aromas, flower elixirs, sounds, crystals and stones. For more detailed information on this I recommend you read his book. His premise is that everything has a vibration, so if you introduce a substance with a particular vibration, it can balance you out overall. For example, he says the colors that are healing frequencies for cancer are blue, blue-violet, and then pink. He says that elixirs for cancer include lilac, amethyst and the fragrances are lilac, sage, and carnation. I did not try these approaches myself, but I suppose it could not hurt to try a fragrance that smells of sage or carnation.

The Law of Attraction

What you are comes to you.

RALPH WALDO EMERSON

According to Wikipedia, The Law of Attraction is the name given to the belief that "like attracts like" and that by focusing on positive or negative thoughts, one can bring about positive or negative results. I put the Law of Attraction under the Spirit section because it's a universal law that we cannot see with the naked eye. My first published book with Simon & Schuster was called *Dating from the Inside Out: How to Use the Law of Attraction in Matters of the Heart*, about dating and the Law of Attraction. It explained how people create the love and relationships they want within themselves before they manifest them out in the world.

According to Baird & Nadel in *Happiness Genes*, your thoughts and emotions affect your body and your magnetic field. They say that EEG tests show your mind's output as a series of electromagnetic waves and your variable heart rate is likewise a measure of your magnetic field. Your magnetic field is an environmental trigger of how your genes behave, and according to these authors, studies prove that you can change your baseline emotional level and thoughts to change your body's measurable magnetic output. This then affects what genes go into action and instruct DNA.

The Law of Attraction says that your magnetic field also directly impacts what you create or attract into your life.

The same principle applies for other things as well. People have a hard time accepting that they may have attracted cancer. I hear you, because I feel like I was pretty happy too. Even from a spiritual perspective, there isn't always a one-to-one correlation because there are so many factors involved, including karma, life habits, environment, genetic predispositions, and even soul lessons that you signed on for before you were incarnated. But having said this, it is still important to look at the Law of Attraction because it can't hurt to do your part to align your thoughts, emotions, and feelings with what you most want to create for your health!

This is not a blame game. Maybe your thoughts are already in alignment with Source and cancer showed up for some other reason. Sometimes the lessons we take on are more for other people's benefit, or an opportunity to deepen our appreciation for life itself.

In her book, *Quantum Success*, Sandra Anne Taylor makes the point that our persistent thoughts create the biggest consequences in our lives. So, look at what thoughts you tell yourself over and over and be sure what you're saying is what you want!

Sometimes The Law of Attraction is actually about trusting that you will get what you want, instead of worrying or perseverating on it. It's the vibration of your thoughts, and the associated emotional vibrations that we emit, which in turn attracts similar vibrations from the cosmic field back to us. So, the action/attraction takes place at an energetic level.

I remembered this when I read *Dying to Be Me* by Anita Moorjani. She advises readers not to chase things but to *allow* them. She says, "Since everything is One, I intend to get what is mine." This is a good Law of Attraction mantra because we draw to us that which we already are.

Moorjani tells the story of how she published the aforementioned book about her cancer experience. She had written a transcript about her near death experience on a related website and a woman saw it and emailed it to author, Wayne Dyer. Wayne Dyer loved the story so much that he mentioned Anita on his radio show and told his publisher. Anita then received an email from a Hay House intern saying if she ever wanted to write a book that they would love to publish it—and she didn't even have an agent! Anita felt she could not have created that situation if she'd tried to plan it. She trusted her Infinite Self and knew that her story would spread in the way that it was meant to.

This is such a great example of creating from trust and essence, and it is a much different experience of manifestation.

I related to Anita's story because my first book, *Dating from the Inside Out*, was published in a similar way. I had written a dating manual for some classes that I was teaching and I sent it out to four publishers without an agent or any publishing experience. Two out of the four publishers called me and were interested. The publisher who I eventually worked with was Cynthia Black, the publisher of *The Secret* and this turned out to be the perfect publishing house of spiritual books. They even had a partnership with Simon and Schuster: Atria Books. So I always felt like the Law of Attraction was at work there because at that time I was allowing things to unfold and was full of confidence and love.

I also took a workshop with author Tama Kieves who self-published her first book: *This Time I Dance*. An editor from Random House spotted it and read it. Keives got an email saying Random House wanted to publish it. Again, no agent or pushing to make it happen.

I've given some examples in the book publishing world about the Law of Attraction but clearly it can be applied in many ways. The Law of Attraction means that you take steps toward what you want *and* you trust and allow things with a similar vibration to be drawn to you.

So, if you want radiant health then you focus on that now by eating well, being active, and noticing all physical improvements. You can praise your body, thank your breath, legs, organs, etcetera for their superb job in sustaining and assisting you. Also you can be aware of the quality of your thoughts regarding your body and health. So for example, if (since your diagnosis) you think, "I am going to die of cancer," or "cancer is going to come back," you can start now to tell yourself instead, "I am radiantly healthy," or "my treatment has banished cancer for good!" Your words create energy and are powerful, so recognize the story that you are vibrating within and choose again if that is not what you intend to create!

To take this process a step further, I want you to realize that your emotions are an important part of the recipe in using The Law of Attraction as a tool. Moorjani learned from her Near Death experience that our emotions are even more powerful than our thoughts, particularly our emotions towards ourselves. So, if you tell yourself, "I am radiantly healthy" but your emotions are extremely fearful, you will not be sending your body a consistent message. So whether you do a love meditation or a visualization to access feelings of peace and love, this will be important in any manifestation process.

I've offered a number of tools to work with your emotions and bring them from fear to love, and to help you work with your thoughts as well. The Law of Attraction calls upon you to bring all these tools to bear so that your thoughts and emotions vibrate love and you are fully open to receive that which you want to receive (and already are).

The reason you imagine yourself having the health you want NOW is because you need to *embody* something in the present in order to attract it. When I wrote my dating book about the Law of Attraction, one of my slogans was, "You attract who you are." Dr. David Hawkins makes this point when he says, "You are attracted to your own energy field, that which you resonate with, that which you have become." So try to envision and feel yourself being peaceful, happy, and healthy, right now.

Another very important point is that you can want something consciously (and affirm this) but unconsciously you are vibrating something else. I wrote about this in depth in *Dating from the Inside Out* around the time *The Secret* came out. As a psychologist, I felt this was my addition to the Law of Attraction philosophy at the time, even though I framed it within the context of dating and relationships. For example, you can say, "All my friends are married and I desperately want to find my soul mate," but if your parents had a miserable marriage then maybe unconsciously you are vibrating, "I need to protect myself and remain alone!"

David Feinstein makes a similar point, saying, "With or without the potency of these interventions, the use of positive images and affirmations is often not effective if there is a contradiction between the person's self-image or core beliefs and the intended changes. When such a contradiction exists, the self-image or core belief tends to prevail." Feinstein suggests that you identify your self-limiting messages and tap on those limiting messages first in order to clear them. In psychotherapy you can talk through those schemas and beliefs to challenge them and replace that self-talk with more positive, adaptive and compassionate beliefs. There are many roads to Rome once you are willing to dig deep and uncover your shadow beliefs about self care, health etcetera.

Bruce Lipton writes that neuroscience now reveals that the subconscious mind is one million times more powerful than the conscious mind and that it runs 95-99% of our behavior. He reminds us that this only allows us to move toward 1-5% of our conscious wishes.

Another way to practice being what you want to manifest, is to give it away. Neale Donald Walsch in his trilogy on *Conversations with God* talks about giving away the things you want. So if you want health, help others be well because what you do to others, you do to yourself. Wanting states the lack of the thing you desire, but giving it away confirms your abundance so you'll get more of it. So how do you give away health? You can give others your faith and conviction of THEIR good health, their recovery/healing being already accomplished, even as their body is still recouperating and share your wisdom about what works for you. Be creative and think of your own way to help people create more health in their lives.

Angels

Every man contemplates an angel in his future self.

Ralph Waldo Emerson

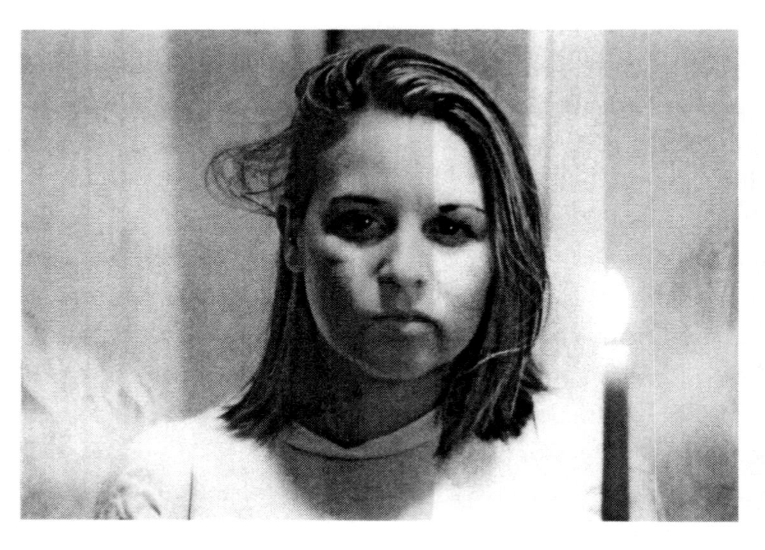

THIS WAS ME AS AN ANGEL ON HALLOWEEN, 8 YEARS AGO

Angels are beings of light who emanate indescribable love and warmth. They are spirit beings mentioned over 250 times in the Bible. They often orchestrate coincidences. In a 1993 Time/CNN poll on angels, 69% of the population believed in angels and 32% had personally felt an angelic presence. A 2011 Associated Press poll revealed that 77% of adults believe these ethereal beings are real. A poll from the Pew Forum on Religion showed that nearly 80% believe in miracles. This surprised me: maybe our society isn't nearly as cynical about angels as I thought!

I always liked the idea of angels, but I never really thought about them in my daily life before being introduced to Chris and being diagnosed with a life-threatening illness. To me, angels are unconditionally loving and comforting and always ready to help without judgment. The thought of having someone or something on your team who exudes love can be helpful when the people in your life are not always so giving.

In his book, *How To Meet and Work with Spirit Guides*, Ted Andrews says that the functions of angels includes praising and attending to the Divine, protecting the faithful, and guiding humanity. The archangels serve as mediators between humanity and the divine powers of the universe.

Also angels have a very high vibration and Chris said that you want to raise your vibration above the energy of cancer so you are like a bug zapper to it. I did not want to talk about fear and symptoms too much, I wanted to remain in a state of love and what better way than to summon angel energy?

Chris said that angels are beings of providence, guidance and protection. During our first session I learned about 7 angels and learned how to invoke what he called "My Angelic Diamond Maitrix" for love and protection. He said I should picture these angels surrounding me like a mercuba or a Star of David. I could invoke this during chemotherapy or whenever I needed a team of angelic help along my cancer path. He said that the angelic maitrix is an energetic container to keep me surrounded in love and light and that it was a higher consciousness than the ordinary consensus reality. He said that everything needs an energetic container. It's funny because when I met Christopher I thought, "When something happens that rocks your world (like cancer) you need a bigger context." I guess the Divine was it!

Dr. Neale (*To Heaven and Back*) says that angels will often push us into a situation that forces our redirection. She says angels told her that without personal trials we would not develop patience or faithfulness. She was told that we each have "personal angels" who guide and watch over us and who very much want us to follow the path that God laid out for us.

In *The War of Art*, Steven Pressman writes, "Angels are agents of evolution . . . Angel midwives congregate around us; they assist us as we give birth to ourselves, to that person we were born to be, to the one whose destiny was encoded in our soul, our daimon, our genius... It makes God happy. Eternity, as Blake might have told us, has opened a portal into time. And we're in it."

The Team of Angelic Helpers I had on this path included:

Archangel Michael: angel of protection and balance. He protects us from lower thoughts and keeps us in Divine mind. He protects us from thoughts that sabotage us and negative emotions and memories and helps us remember to turn them over to God. He provides a shield of love to catch our negative thoughts about ourselves and others and he returns it to Source. It's like game of catch that you can play, of catching your negative emotions and thoughts so they don't influence your body or decisions. He catches all shames, blames, and comparisons and holds you only in love in the present moment.

Archangel Gabriel: angel for clarity of perception and insight who could show me the benefits of cancer and would help me come through this experience stronger and would help my 22 books come from Spirit. He guides our intuition and can hold us in the light.

Archangel Raphael: Supports and heals our physical bodies bringing healing into our glands, cells, and endocrine system.

Archangel Uriel: Angel who is the strength of God. He holds our mental body in love and is a container of goodness against the darkness around us and helps us maintain boundaries to protect all 4 energetic bodies.

Archangel Ariel: Angel of joy who would allow me to receive and allow joy because cancer is the energy of misery and it shrinks from joy.

Metatron: Angel at the throne of creation who opens the corridor from heaven to earth and allows us to be vessels of love and light and lets this flow to all four energy bodies.

Sandalphson: Angel of the root chakra who opens a corridor to Mother Earth energy.

Thank you to my angels!

If you love angels, I'd recommend you watch some movies about them. Here are a number of movies that you can rent: *Date With an Angel*, *City of Angels*, *Heaven Only Knows*, *I Married an Angel*, *Michael*, *Dogma*, *Gabriel*, *Faraway, So Close*, and *A Life Less Ordinary*.

Besides thinking of Divine Angels coming to save us in our time of need, we can remember that there is an earth angel in every one of us and we can look to find that love and radiance in ourselves and each other on a daily basis.

Anyway, during my treatment I surrounded myself with Angels in one way or another. My sister Avra sent me a care package with a bunch of little cardboard angel cutouts for my daughter Sera (whose crib is in our room) and I stuck them all around, in plants, on candles and on my bookshelves. See the following page.

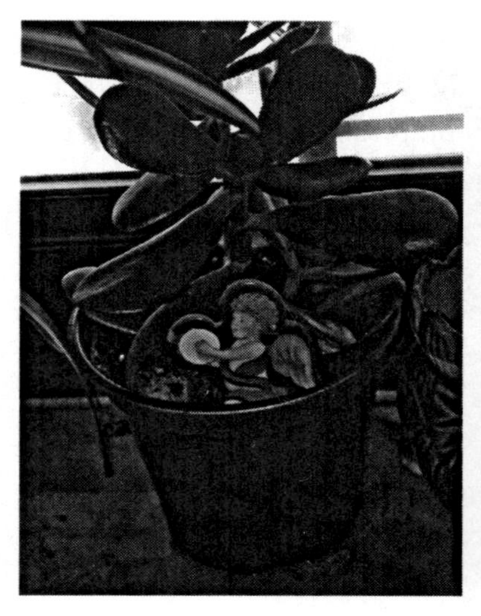
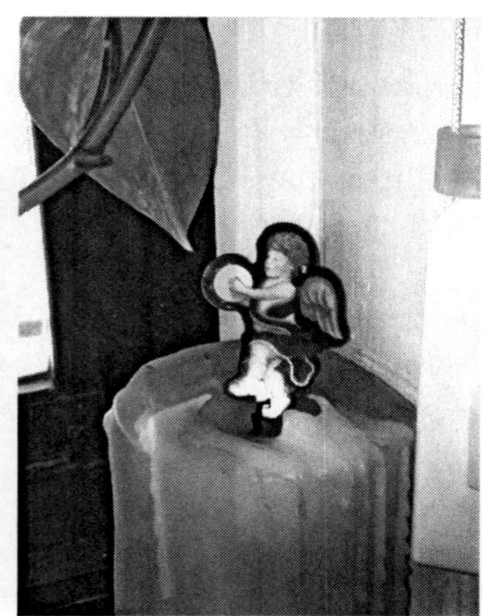

I also listened to my angel meditation at night.

I even made a visual representation of my Divine Angelic Maitrix so I could remember how my angels surround me at any time and could summon them. Maybe you want to do the same. My drawing is on the following page.

Later on my cancer path, Christopher told me that I had advanced Spiritually, and now he sensed the Angels of the Shekhinah around me, above my crown, which he said was like an initiation and graduation. I had always loved the Shekhinah, the Jewish vision of the Feminine Divine, who was said to preside at the wailing wall and who was also the Sabbath bride. Chris said these angels had light that was golden, purple, silver and white, like the aurora borealis. I had even more support around me now and he said I can add to my prayers, "Above my head, above my head, the Holy Shekhinah." He told me that we do not get to a spiritual place like this without hardship. He said that the lives in which we struggle often have the biggest spiritual breakthroughs and are how we can be of the most help to others. He reminded me that St. Francis was in physical pain but he radiated emotional joy

My Healing Temple

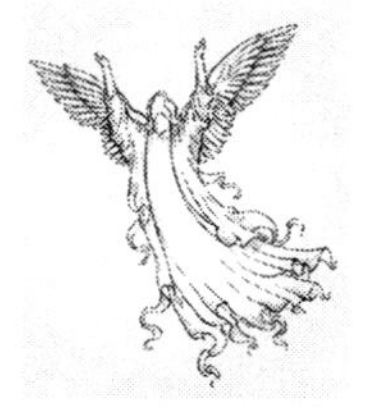

Metratron
Golden corridor to align with Source

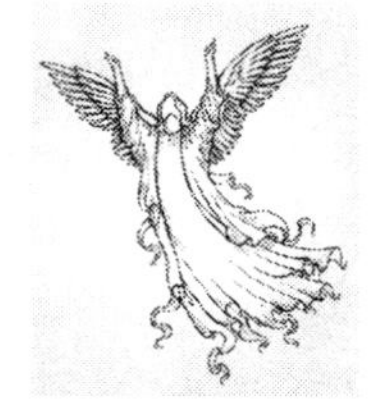

Archangel Michael
Protection

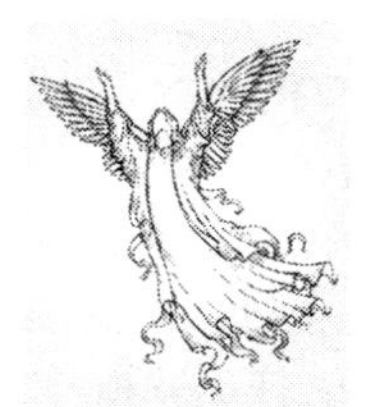

Archangel Ariel
Joyful creation in my heart

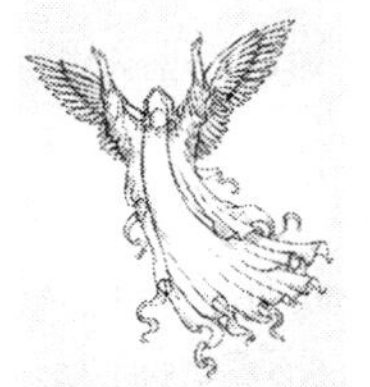

Archangel Gabriel
Insight

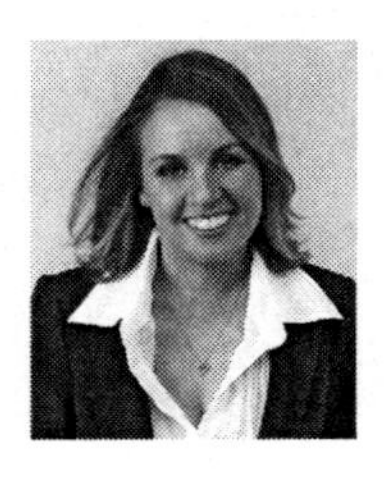

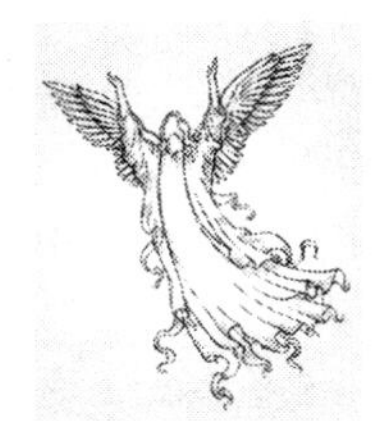

Archangel Raphael
Healing

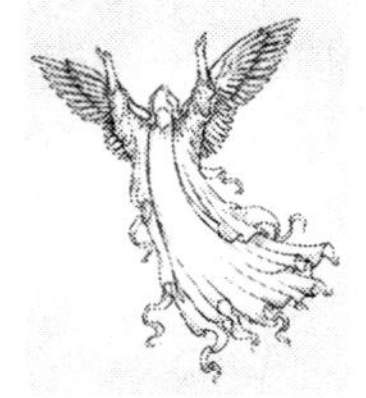

Archangel Sandalfson
Expands my Root Chakra

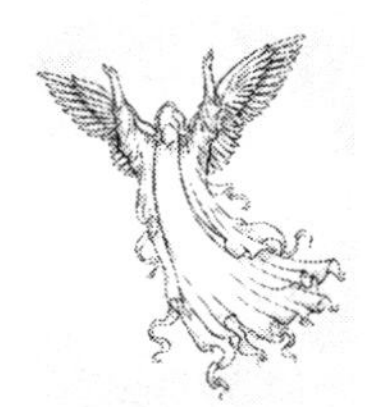

Archangel Uriel
Merging heart and head

because he wasn't body identified. Every experience of suffering is a teacher or a hurdle and if we let them, the angels and ascended masters can lift us over our obstacles. Chris quoted a Japanese saying:

Life has suffering.
Suffering brings pain.
Pain makes man think.
Thinking makes man wise.
Acting on wisdom leads to enlightenment.
Then from enlightenment comes joy.

Ask yourself when you might have experienced the guidance or help of your guardian angel. I'm not sure if it was angels intervening, but a few instances of synchronicity or Divine providence do come to mind. The first was when I was in graduate school doing my dissertation on Holocaust survivors. I went to the library at the Holocaust museum in Washington, DC and while I was there, I asked the librarian there if they had any photo books on a small town called Chotin in Bessarabia. This is where my maternal grandfather was from, but I had never met him because he was killed in the Holocaust when my mother was three. Much to my surprise the librarian brought out a book that had one picture with him in it. I made a photocopy and my mother (who had been 3 when he was killed) saw her father for the first time (when she was 60). This seemed like an act of Providence. The other instance was when I was in a car crash, and a strange man suddenly appeared to call the police, to get me out of my car and to make sure that I had my cell phone with me, and then he suddenly disappeared.

Ask yourself, have you have any moments like these? Are you open to signs from your Guardian angels?

Doreen Virtue suggests we talk to our guardian angels and ask them for help. We can notice signs, like when things repeat themselves, and then we can ask our angels for clarification.

I bought a painting of an angel and hung it in my office. I suggest putting statues or pictures of angels around to remind you of their loving, healing energy. Here is the picture of the angel in my office:

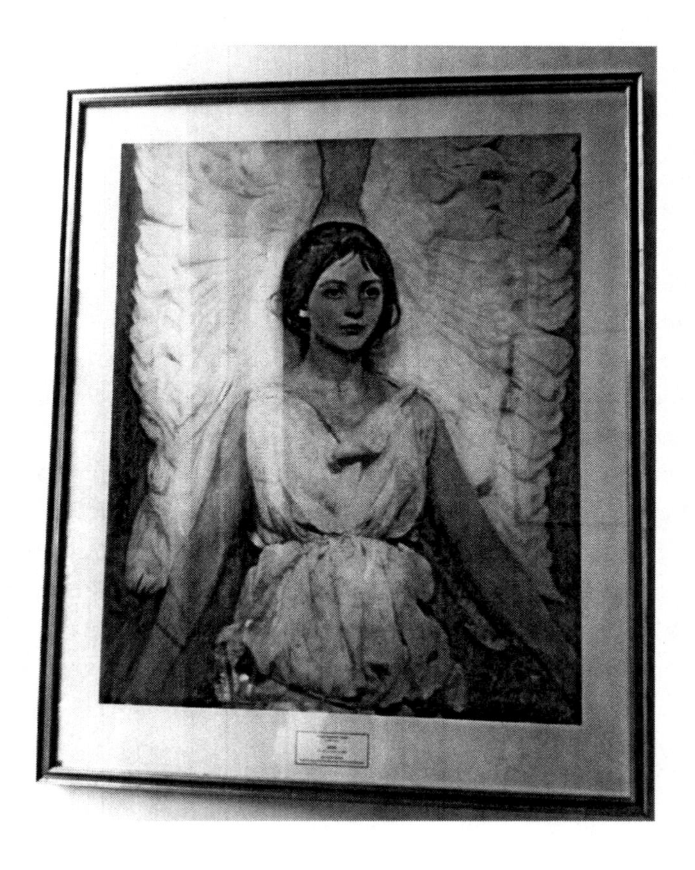

Some people also use Angel Oracle cards to get angelic messages. Some decks to consider playing with are: *Archangel Oracle Cards*, *Magical Messages for the Fairies* and *Messages from Your Angels*, by Doreen Virtue.

Cellular Healing

From a cymatic or vibratory standpoint, disharmony is disease. The critical concept to grasp here is that all manifestations of disease, whether diagnosed as 'physiological' or 'psychological,' result from disruption (in the form of toxicity or trauma) of the primary electromagnetic harmonies and rhythms contained in the auric fields and corresponding chakras . . . These bioenergy centers have an intimate relationship with DNA that gives them direct regulatory access to all cellular functions. Therefore, if we can find a way to reset our bioenergy blueprint through harmonic resonance, we can go directly to the root of disease processes.

Sol Luckman

In *Quantum Healing*, Deepak Chopra says all of us have memories inside our cells. These memories within our degenerative cells are passed on and replicate. Chopra found that survivors of serious disease did two things. They got in touch with their body's infinite intelligence, and accessed the cell memory and let it go. Chopra calls that process Cellular Healing. Chopra writes, "The immune system knows all our secrets, all our sorrows . . . it knows every moment a cancer patient spends in the light of life or in the shadow of death, because it turns those moments into the body's physical reality."

Joyce Hawkes wrote a book called *Cell-Level Healing*, which discusses how healing energy can affect cells. Hawke was a biophysicist and a fellow at the Advancement of Science. After a near death experience, she explored indigenous healing practices and transitioned from a cellular scientist to a cell-level healer. She says there are 100 trillion cells in our body and she reminds us that 96% of the universe is beyond our view because it is not in the visible spectrum. Hawkes says that many factors can contribute to illness including emotional trauma, genetics, stress, and environmental toxins. She even says that limiting beliefs can cause blockages. Hawkes reaches into the body energetically to promote cellular healing. She says energy flow is key and writes that when disease prevents large areas of flow in a critical organ, the whole body dies.

Hawkes says that cancer cells are part of our body and that if a cell of any tissue type divides too fast and at random, it may result in a tumor. She says that an enzyme called p53 regulates the timetable for cell division in normal cells. Cancer cells lack the p53 enzymes and are strangely embryonic in structure. Hawkes recommends that patients do meditations to affirm cell balance and to ask your cells to synthesize p53 for proper cell growth rates. She describes this in more depth in her book, along with a story of shrinking a tumor for a woman with breast cancer. She offers healing sessions and I will put her website in Appendix C.

Our Energy Body

The ultimate approach to healing will be to remove the abnormalities at the subtle-energy level which led to the manifestation of illness in the first place.

DR. RICHARD GERBER

Everything in life is vibration and the human energy fields include sound, magnetic, light, electrical, thermal, and electromagnetic fields, accord to Ted Andrews. He says that in Western philosophy we have 4 subtle bodies that make up our human energy: physical, emotional (astral), mental and spiritual, and for the greatest health they must all be aligned.

Energy Medicine describes the growing perspective of the body as a system of energies and applies this understanding to promote healing and health. Dr. Mehmet Oz, one of the most well known and respected surgeons in the U.S. announced that "the next frontier in medicine is energy medicine." Carolyn Myss, author and medical intuitive said, "the belief that repressing an illness through drugs is of use will come to be seen as harmful rather than beneficial." And Dr. David Hawkins says, "The energy field of that which we truly are is ever present and gives us an intense sense of aliveness when we let go of the obstacles."

A great book about our energetic system and how to remove obstacles in our energy is *Energy Medicine* by Donna Eden. She can see energy and she says that everyone has a different physical structure and energy anatomy, but there are still useful tools and energy principles that we can all use and benefit from. She even says that energy medicine can help you prepare for surgery, can be used with medical treatments, and can help with side effects from chemotherapy and medications. Her book contains more than 100 procedures to help the energy in your body flow and heal. She talks about the power of self-care in energy medicine.

Energy Medicine describes our energy system in terms of the chakras, meridians, aura, radiant circuits and more. Eden says that matter follows energy and when your energy is vibrant, so is your body. Chronically marshalling extra energy for the immune or fight-or-flight response tends to undermine your overall health and vitality and Eden's book gives techniques to shift harmful energy patterns that have grown out of our stress-filled environments. She explains that it's much wiser to treat the imbalance while it is still only a disturbance in the energy field than to wait until it has progressed into a physical symptom that is far more traumatic and entrenched. She tells us that our energy body holds the blueprint of our physical body's health so it's important we learn to understand it and work with it: "Energy medicine draws on the principle that by establishing greater teamwork among body, mind and spirit, you can transcend the automated strategies designed by evolution."

Deepak Chopra discusses how energy affects our body, saying, "Drugs, too, are bundles of energy and the effects they cause in your body (including side effects) are nothing but energy patterns moving one way, instead of another." He even discusses cancer specifically, saying, "It only takes a seed of disruption, such as a malignant cell, to spread incoherence everywhere; if the seed is allowed to grow, the energy of the whole body will break down. It may sound strange to think of cancer as distorted energy, but that's what it is . . . dealing with your own energy is the most effortless way to heal yourself, because you are going directly to the source. When a distorted energy pattern returns to normal, the problem disappears."

The idea is to get stuck energy flowing again. Energy can be stuck from limiting beliefs, stuck emotions, or for physical reasons. Chopra advises, "Turn entropy into evolution." This is a great healing mantra in all areas of body, mind, emotions and Spirit. If we can learn about where we are stuck energetically, we can remove the barrier and restore the flow, thereby learning about ourselves and growing in wisdom and maturity.

Donna Eden offers a 5-minute daily energy routine (on pg 72) of her book *Energy Medicine* to enforce positive energy habits and she has an Energy Medicine Kit which includes a DVD of these techniques on her website: www.innersource.net. She says that this short routine can make you more resilient against illness and stress.

Auras

The human aura is the energy field that surrounds the physical body in all directions. It is three-dimensional. . . . The stronger and more vibrant our auric field is, the easier it is for us to attune to all the subtle influences in our life—including our spirit guides.

TED ANDREWS

Everyone is surrounded by a colored hue called an aura. Eden describes it as a multi-dimensional sphere of energy that emanates from your body and interacts with the Earth's atmosphere. She says that the aura is protective and filters energies, drawing in what we need. When you are sick your aura will often collapse in to protect you.

For over 20 years, experiments on the human aura have been performed in Valerie Hunt's Energy Field's Laboratory at UCLA. In the experiments, aura readings were compared with neurophysiological measures and the colors seen by 8 aura readers corresponded with each other and exactly with electromyograph (EMG) wave patterns picked up by electrodes on the skin at the observed spot. Experiments have also shown that auras shift with acupuncture, prayer, and changes in thought.

Donna Eden says the aura has 7 layers and corresponds with the chakras. Eden says that she sees the first band of the aura as the energetic double of our physical body and it's critical for our survival. When energy imbalances in your body become too excessive the aura can't protect us and it becomes thin, disorganized, or collapsed. Auric disturbances can lead to health problems, including leaks and tears, too many toxic energies, and chronic collapse and stagnation, and it can become locked into an unhealthy state. Eden teaches the technique of "The Hook-Up"—how to clear and strengthen your chakras by scanning, shifting, fluffing and weaving your aura to rejuvenate it.

Author and psychic Michelle Whitedove says every living being has a soul and an aura, which is the energy field radiating from the soul. According to her, gifted psychics can read the energy from an aura and determine a soul's ranking, past lives, and history. She says that plants, trees and even rocks have an aura!

I intuitively understand auras but I have not yet seen one myself. Once, a long time ago, I took a Reiki certification class and was able to see energy like little bubbles moving through the air, but I do not yet have the ability to see colors of energy. Fascinated to learn about this, I recently read a book called *Change Your Aura, Change Your Life* by Barbara Martin and Dimitri Moralis which I would recommend if you want to explore auras and chakra healing.

According to the aforementioned authors everything has an auric field, until it dies. The aura is a spiritual reservoir of energy and each auric color is there for a reason. The aura radiates a spiritual energy that's reflective of everything you feel, think and do: it reflects your strengths, weaknesses, soul's purpose and character. What's especially exciting about Barbara and Dimitri's book (besides describing the aura in such detail) is that they explain how to change your aura by drawing in new colors of Divine light, so that you can then change your life. They also point out that the more light you are able to draw in, the higher your consciousness, so that too is a good motivation for working with auras. So, for example, if you want prosperity, you can do their meditations and draw in turquoise light. There are many more examples of how to work on forgiveness, fear, career, anger, and so forth.

In *Energy Medicine*, Donna Eden says that an easy way to restore your energy is to fill your bathtub with baking soda to cleanse your aura. You can hold the neurovascular points on your forehead for a minute while bathing. This is explained further in her book.

The psychic John Holland discusses the importance of color in people's auras. Here's what he says about the colors he sees in people's auras and what they can often mean:

Red: these people have power and are often physical.

Orange: these people are often happy.

Yellow: these people are often friendly and sensitive.

Green: these people are often being healed or are healers.

Blue: these people are often spiritual and can be psychic.

Indigo: these people have imagination and can be gurus.

Violet: these people have higher wisdom, creativity and enlightenment.

White: these people emanate truth, purity and innocence.

Brown: These people often work with gardening and the earth.

Black: Could mean illness or could be protective.

Gold: This can mean protection and spirituality.

Pink: These people have no mask. The pink color can make things calm.

I learned more about colors from Ted Andrews in his book, *How to Heal With Color*. He explains that color is light broken down into different wavelengths and therefore, colors. He says that different frequencies of light affect different energies of the body. The human body has different energy fields and certain colors can restore balance.

White: is strengthening, purifying and balancing.

Black: can be protective.

Red: activates our physical life force and deeper passions.

Orange: activates joy, wisdom, sociability and emotions.

Yellow: stimulates our mind and confidence.

Green: balances energy, hope, faith and peace but it helps things grow so it should not be used on tumors!

Blue: relaxing to our system and awakens intuition.

Indigo: healing spiritual color, detoxifies and can awaken intuition and devotion.

Violet: activates the crown chakra and is good to use on the cancerous conditions of the body

Pink: awakens love and compassion and stimulates the immune system.

Purple: purifies the system and shrinks things, like tumors.

Andrews suggests that we meditate and breathe these colors in.

I did not try using color during my healing process (beyond doing my chakra meditations) but I would be interested if any of you try this and find it helpful. My Bibliography will include a few books on this for you to read as a starting point.

Our Dreams Can Be Messengers

Man is a genius when he is dreaming.

KUROSAWA

Our dreams can give us messages and let us know what we need to pay attention to. Many famous inventions were inspired by dreams. For example, Elias Howe invented the sewing machine based upon an inspiring dream. Descartes said dreams revealed his new philosophy of science. James Watson had a dream of a spiral staircase that helped him discover the structure of DNA, and Paul McCartney dreamed the melody to "Yesterday." I'm sure there are many more examples. Have you ever received wisdom or a problem or a foreshadowing of events in your dreams?

I am not a developed psychic but there have been times that my subconscious has tried to alert me to things. For instance, a week or two before 911 I had a dream and when I woke up, this poem came to me *whole.* I jotted it all down on a paper by my bed with my eyes closed and later typed it up. For me it symbolized the catastrophe sparked by differences, which resulted in people jumping off the World Trade Center as it crumbled. Here was that poem:

My Borders Grow

As I grow
My Borders grow
Encompassing
More territory

All the gravel and dirt
Mountains and valleys
A skyscraper
And a lone tree

I take in all
That surrounds me

I reach out
To touch the hands
Of those I didn't think
I wanted to know

And as I do
My borders grow

More light
Can filter in
More darkness too

And when I'm lost
I reach for You

Love eventually
Has no bounds

The borders
Go deep underground
And contain it all

So don't be afraid
To catch a falling few

Next year
You'll turn around,
and they'll be catching you.

* * *

Although the above poem could not have warned me about the event to come (and maybe it wasn't a foreshadowing of events) it was an accurate commentary about what may have caused it and hopefully we can all learn the necessary spiritual lessons going forward.

During my cancer experience, much of this book was written from thoughts I got in my sleep. In fact, the entire introduction was scrawled in pencil on some scrap paper during twilight state at 3 a.m. while I was in bed. I feel that we have access to more information in that state of consciousness than we realize.

Recently, I had a dream about a rattlesnake. When I looked up the symbolic meaning of snakes, it was often interpreted as symbolizing transformation and kundalini energy. It can also symbolize the caduceus symbol of healing. In a section on animal totems in Michelle Whitedove's book, *She Talks with Angels*, she describes the snake as a symbol of transmutation, the sexual and spiritual energy that comes from kundalini energy. She says it represents healing energy and magical gifts.

Pay attention to your dreams and write them down as you are on your cancer path. Ask for wisdom before you go to sleep and keep a pen and paper by your bedside. Keep your eyes half- closed while you write so you don't switch into your waking state of consciousness.

Once you identify your dream symbols you can look them up online or elsewhere to discern the meanings associated with them. There is also a great book called *Animal Speaks* by Ted Andrews that richly explores animal symbolism. See Resources.

DREAM EXERCISE

Keep a journal by your bed. When you wake up record any symbols or dream fragments you remember. Free associate to how you are feeling in the dream, or draw pictures if that is easier for you. You can look up any symbols in a dream dictionary and think about how your unconscious or Spirit might be trying to guide you. This process will give you access to other parts of yourself.

Symbols, Signs, & Mystical Experiences

Spirit communicates through synchronicities, signs and our dreams . . . Synchronicities are what some people call coincidences . . . everything happens for a reason . . . review the event and try to see the message.

MICHELLE WHITEDOVE

During my treatment process I found that a few healing symbols kept popping up for me. When I saw them on my journey it was just a reminder that spirit was with me, guiding me. I will tell you about a couple of my special symbols here with the hope that you will likewise journal and discover your special symbols and will be inspired by life's little surprises and the universe's ways of reminding you that you are never alone.

Deepak Chopra says, "External guidance comes to people for whom the best proof of Spirit is physical." In *To Heaven and Back*, Dr. Neale says that God's messengers are everywhere and they come to us in forms we can accept, like an owl or a human. She tells a story about the death of her son. He was hit by a car at a location that had wild Alpine pink roses, far from her house. One day she was walking her property looking for the right spot to create a garden in her son's memory. She found pink-colored blossoms of wild Alpine roses which were the exact color, shape, and appearance of those that were in the field where her son died. She had never seen the blossoms before her son's death, and had definitely never seen them on her property, so she knew it was a sign from her son. She invites readers to keep a 6-12 month journal of coincidences, which I think is a great idea. She says to write major events, the circumstances, and how things fell into place. In addition, or alternatively, she suggest you make note of the times when you've struggled—when bad things that have happened and what happened as a result. When you look back in your journal, you will see how people, events, and outcomes were interconnected. Paying attention to "coincidences" and symbols will strengthen your intuitive intelligence and awareness of this invisible reality.

FEATHERS & ANGEL WINGS

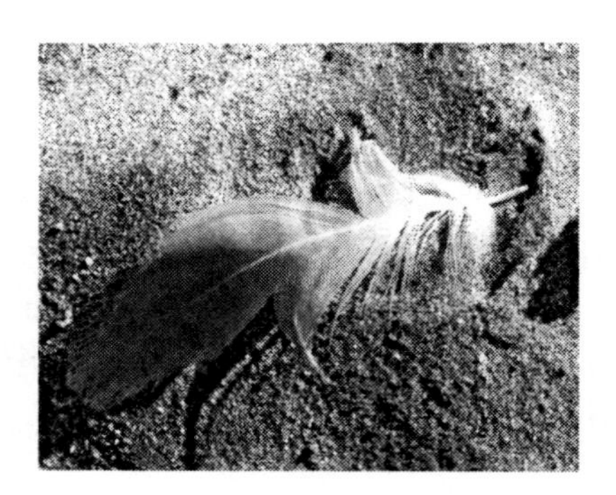

I tried to walk the beach a few times a week during my treatment. Often I would look down and see a white feather and stick it in my pocket or purse. It was probably just a seagull feather but to me it was a reminder that my angels were with me and this made me smile.

A RAINBOW

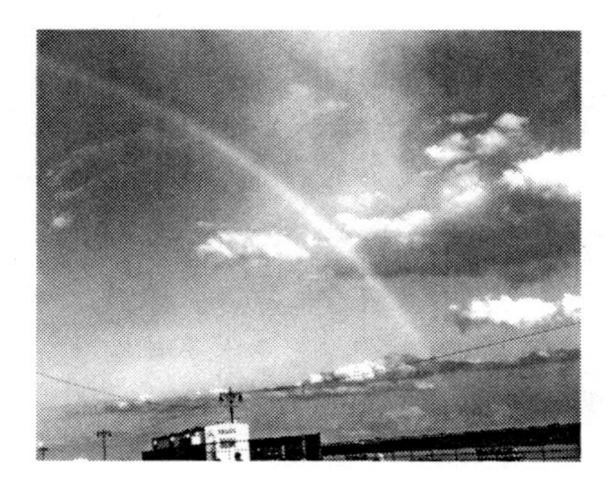

One day during my treatment we were driving in our van with my kids and my husband and a huge rainbow spread out right before us. It was drizzling a bit but the rainbow seemed to form out of the blue. I took this as a sign that everything was going to be alright. Ted Andrews says that rainbows represent opportunities to heal and be healed, and harkening back to color therapy, a rainbow contains all colors to strengthen all systems: body, mind, heart, and Spirit.

LAVENDER WISTERIA

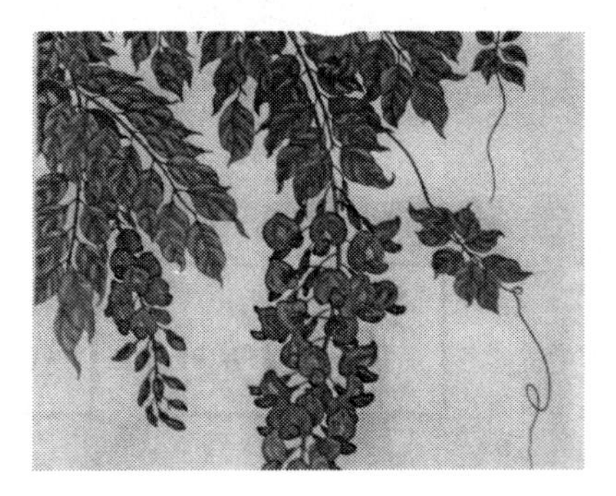

Lavender wisteria has long been my favorite flower and you don't see it everywhere! So when I do see it, it is like a wink from the universe and my angels. I looked up the meaning of lavender wisteria. It seems to be a symbol of humility and reflection in Shin Buddhism. It symbolizes thoughtful reverence and a need for peace, quiet, and an honoring of our divine essence. It can also mean endurance in the face of heartache, steadfastness, and creative expansion and spontaneity.

I have seen lavender wisteria so many places since I started treatment—in the park where I get off the subway, near my house, and then I noticed this painting titled "Lavender Wisteria" when I was sitting in my radiology oncologist's waiting room. The signs are everywhere if you look for them!

If I am driving somewhere and see a random tree or vines of lavender wisteria I know my angels are telling me I am on the right path.

LADYBUGS

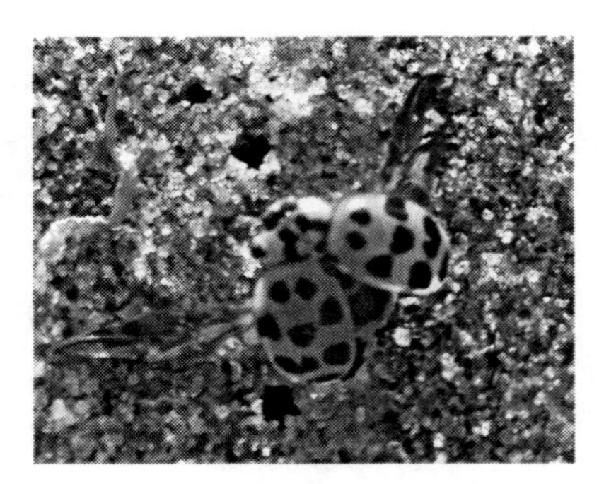

LADYBUGS MAKING LOVE

This is a fun one. I live near the beach and as I've said I walk there frequently. Well, I don't know a lot about ladybugs but I will tell you that I didn't know they loved the beach too! When I was going through my treatment I saw 2 ladybugs making love, I saw ladybugs everywhere in the sand (and had to be careful not to step on any), and even saw one with lots of spots crawling on our van.

I guess most people know that ladybugs mean good luck according to folklore. Other meanings associated with the ladybug include protection, abundance, delight, and trust. Some say the ladybug reminds us that life is short so we should let go of worries and enjoy life to the fullest. And while you may not take such "signs" seriously, just noticing such love and luck-filled notions will make you feel good when you are on a difficult journey.

So, look for signs in your life that good things will be revealed to you in time and little reminders that Spirit is with you.

THE BEACH, OCEAN & NATURE

And my shells? I can sweep them all into my pocket. They are only there to remind me that the sea recedes and returns eternally.

ANNE MORROW LINDBERG

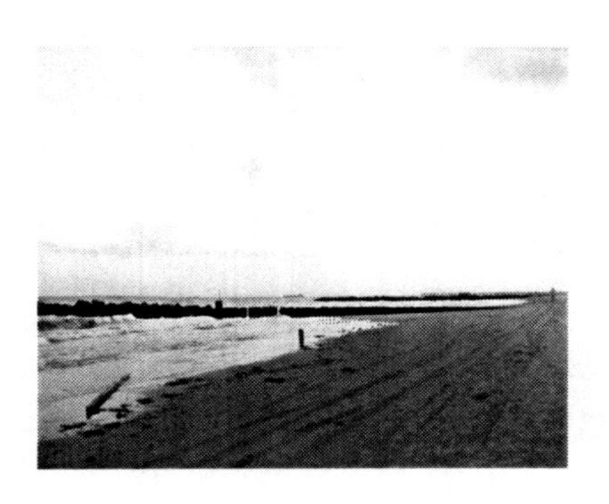

Before I was diagnosed with breast cancer we were seriously considering buying a house in Merrick, Long Island. Afterwards, I was so glad to have had the beach near me during this healing process. Nature in general is very healing, but to me the ocean represents the Great Mother. I felt surrounded by love and peace when I would walk there and I felt particularly lucky to have it at my doorstep. I would hope that most of you have a park or some magical space with a stream of water or trees close by. Otherwise, you can find a spot that brings you nourishment and calm, and make the effort to go there. For example, a 30-minute train ride would take me to the Brooklyn Botanical Gardens, or a one-hour train ride gets me to the beach in Rockaway. What's important is that spending some time alone in nature is vastly healing.

In *The Nature-Speak Oracle*, Ted Andrews says that the beach is a mystical place; the doorway to Spirit. It means that you are on track for balance and healing. All the primal elements of nature come together there—fire, earth, air and water.

BUTTERFLIES

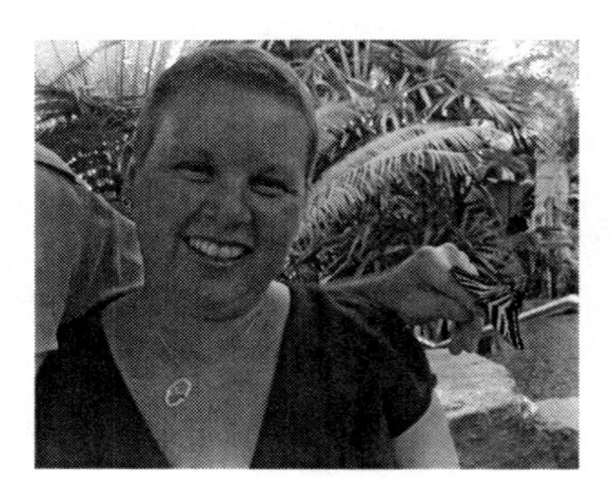

I love butterflies. To me they symbolize transformation. We went to a Butterfly Conservatory and I saw a sign in the gift shop. It sounded like butterfly wisdom: *"True Happiness is like the Butterfly. The more you pursue it, the more it will elude you, but if you are patient and still it will come softly and land on your shoulders."*

Butterflies are symbols of the soul and transformation. When I googled the symbolism of butterflies much of what was said resonated with me. Here's what I found: "Butterflies unquestionably embrace the chances of her environment and body, represent faith, transition, celebration, lightness and joy. It means that growth and change does not have to be traumatic and that you can let go of old behavior and transform in to the next major life change."

Michelle Whitedove says that butterflies represent a change of state, a transformation, and a journey of the soul.

THE LABYRINTH

It was very empowering for me to see life not as a series of ups and downs, but as a spiral in which even as you are moving down you are still moving forward.

ARIANNA HUFFINGTON

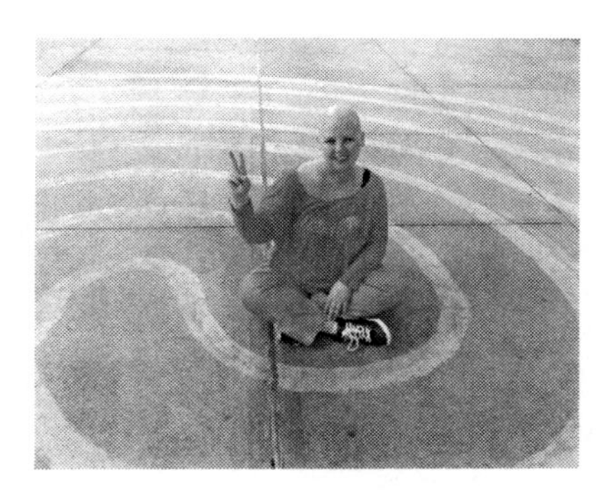

To me a labyrinth is a good symbol for the Cancer Path. It symbolizes a journey to our sacred center, our heart. Other symbolism of the labyrinth includes: royal power, rebirth, initiation, body/mind/spirit, a sacred center, wholeness, going with the flow and having faith. Christopher added that the labyrinth is what happens when we are headed to our healing center and we take wrong turns to go back out again. We may sometimes be making progress yet it doesn't seem like it. Sometimes it's 2 steps forward, one step back, but we're still making progress.

I had a vision of a labyrinth for my book cover and as a result, I also put a labyrinth design for my henna crown. My friend Rachel and I found a labyrinth in the village in NYC and walked it. It was very centering and felt like I was finding my way to my Higher self. My family also went to the labyrinth in Battery Park during my treatment.

There are labyrinths many places that you can visit. There is a famous labyrinth in the Grace Cathedral. In Greek mythology, the labyrinth was designed by Daedalus to imprison the Minotaur, but the labyrinth serves a symbolic meaning, as well. "Walking the labyrinth" is said to be a deeply personal and revealing meditative experience by which a person gains insights into their true nature." Try this out and see what the experience does for you. It will remind you that all the twists and turns will ultimately lead you back to Source.

Prayer

Let us be silent that we may hear the whisper of God.

RALPH WALDO EMERSON

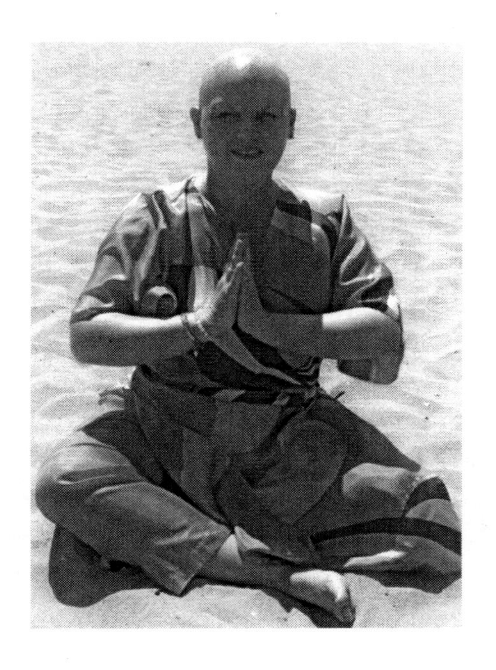

I always prayed but since cancer it became a daily event. Research has shown that prayer has healing effects and evokes a high level of consciousness. An analysis of 43 studies on people with advanced cancer revealed that people who reported spiritual well-being coped more effectively with terminal illnesses and found meaning in their experience.

Dr. David Hawkins says that devotional acts like prayer calibrate at the same level as joy. Author and psychic Michelle Whitedove says that prayers are powerful but they must be said with faith and gratitude. In *Conversations With God Volume 3*, Neale Donald Walsh says that the highest form of prayer is thought control. Our every thought is considered a prayer because they are requests to the universe so we need to try and make them positive.

It has been reported that 4 billion people have no religious beliefs but I don't know if this means they do not believe in God as well. Although I am not religious in a traditional sense, I believe in God and for me prayer is helpful. It is wonderful to think that through prayer you can speak into eternity and find a resonant echo in challenging events, along with a powerful, ever-present compassion. Studies done on the impact of prayer and spirituality have mixed results.

The U.S. Office of Technology Assessment reported that a survey of articles published in the *Journal of Family Practice* over ten years found that 83% of studies on "religiosity" found a positive effect on physical health. (Religiosity was measured by participation in religious ceremony, social support, prayer, and belief in a higher being.)

Another study of two psychiatric journals over 12 years found that for the studies that measured religiosity, 92% showed a benefit for mental health, 4% were neutral, and 4% showed harm.

In the late 1980s, a study in San Francisco found that heart patients who were prayed for by others appeared to have fewer complications, although length of hospital stay and death rates did not differ between those who were prayed for and those who were not. A larger study at a Kansas City hospital coronary care unit reported similar findings. Although overall length of hospital stay and time in the critical care unit did not differ between groups, the group that had been prayed for had 11% fewer complications. These results suggested that prayer might be helpful when used with conventional medical care, although more research was needed. When a research group reanalyzed 14 of these studies, they concluded that intercessory prayer had no effect on any medical outcomes.

A group of Harvard researchers studied more than 1,800 patients who were undergoing heart surgery in 2006. The patients were randomly assigned to 3 groups. The first group was told that prayers would be said for them, while the second and third groups were told that they might or might not have prayers said for them. The first and second groups received prayer, and the third group did not. Complications occurred within 30 days for 59% of the first group, 52% of the second group, and 51% of the third group. Prayer did not reduce complications for those who had heart surgery in this large, well-controlled scientific study. So at this point scientific evidence does not support claims of reduced complications in those who receive prayer.

In *Prayer is Good Medicine*, by Larry Dossey, he describes why it's good for doctors to pray for their patients. He says that over 90% of women and over 80% of men pray regularly—and interestingly, he mentions that surveys show that 75% of patients believe that their physicians should address spiritual issues as part of their medical care and 50% want their doctor to pray for them! (That last part surprised me!) Here's something that surprised me further: according to Dr. David Larson at the National Institute for Healthcare Research in MD, 43% of American physicians do pray for their patients! So, perhaps my perception or limited experience of doctors as being often overly scientific to the exclusion of the patient's heart, mind, and spirit isn't entirely accurate.

Larry Dossey also says that in 1996 one-third of medical schools had alternative medicine courses and five medical schools had programs dedicated to the relationship between faith and health. He says the research shows that praying regularly is 80% beneficial in terms of preventing and coping with illness. Spindrift is an organization that has studied the positive effects of prayer—so clearly the tides are slowly beginning to turn.

Others may not feel prayer has magical or spiritual effects on illness but they admit that it can affect health by initiating a relaxation response, similar to that of meditation. In the 1970s Dr. Herbert Benson at Harvard Medical School studied how the body responded to Christian prayer, biofeedback, hypnosis, and relaxation techniques, and he discovered that with each the body showed a relaxation response consisting of lowered heart rate, blood pressure, and breathing rate, a reduced need for oxygen, and less carbon dioxide production.

Again, I am not pushing that prayer will cure all illness, I just would like the power of alternative healing practices to be open to discussion and research so that such healing methods could augment healing instead of being met with immediate derision.

In *Prayer is Good Medicine*, Dr. Larry Dossey tells a story about Peregrine Laziosi, a Catholic priest who lived in Italy from 1260-1345. Peregrine developed advanced cancer of his foot and was scheduled for an amputation. He prayed before sleeping that healing would come to him in the night and had a vision that he was cured. When he awoke the cancer was gone, surgery was cancelled, and he spent his life ministering to people with cancer. He was canonized as St. Peregrine in 1726 and he is known as the patron saint of cancer patients.

While I love the above story (and I wonder if the level of conviction affects the results of prayer), I am one who at the moment, hedges my bets. I prefer to do the standard medical treatment and pray. I fully believe miracles are possible, I just don't know if they are probable. My approach is that praying can't hurt and it could help, so why not do it?

A Course in Miracles

There are only two ways to live your life. One is as though nothing is a miracle. The other is as though everything is a miracle.

Albert Einstein

I had my cancer yoga class on Tuesdays after work in Union Square and then I had a little window of time before my husband picked me up. I wanted to use that time well and I'd always wanted to learn about A Course in Miracles. Many of the spiritual psychology authors I liked practiced this philosophy but I found the book hard to understand on my own, so I had long wanted a teacher but hadn't had time to find one. I fortuitously found a Course in Miracles class being held at a center called CRS right near my yoga class. It turned out the class was at a different time, but I was able to meet up with a woman from the class named Kathleen for an hour each week at a coffee shop downstairs from the center for a nominal fee. I was so happy it was something I could afford and I would finally be learning this material.

During our first lesson we discussed the idea that there was love and there was fear—and that we are love, but we have forgotten this. We explored these two dichotomies: Love is Spirit and oneness and fear comes from ego, the body, and being separate. We discussed how any experience is an invitation to love. We discussed how we are of Spirit and not the body and how this world is an illusion that isn't real. This reminds us that we can engage in conflict or we can accept peace and joy in every situation and be like our Source.

We explored the dichotomy of acting versus reacting, and how to see every person as perfect and a child of God. She suggested we view every person and situation as non-threatening and helpful. Kathleen said that everything is either an expression of love or a call for love, and that people want to be accepted and whole. She went even further, saying that there are no "other" people and others merely reflect your mind back to you. The ego's nature is to like conflict and separation but Spirit only knows love, so we can choose. We do not have to operate from the standpoint of protection. If you have everything you need there is no lack and you can be defenseless with others, which is an extremely powerful position.

The idea is to be in peace all the time, but we can't do this alone. We can ask God for help as a bridge between these two worlds. We need to realize that it's not up to us to fix things, it's up to God. You can also trust and choose peace no matter what is happening or what the outcome is. Our emotions are a byproduct of our thoughts, so if we feel anger, sadness, or worry we are coming from thoughts of fear and not love. The healing is learning to see others as perfect through the eyes of love.

We can turn down the ego and see that Spirit is always there. We need stillness of the body and mind in order to hear God. This made ponder why I have not been getting more regular messages before diagnosis. I am always rushing around. It might be like God is calling but she always gets a busy signal. I need to create periods of surrender, emptiness, and stillness so God can come more fully into my life and heart.

Kathleen told me to start by just observing my feelings and trying not to limit my peace. When I left I told her I really wanted to learn how to apply these principles to everyday conflicts and situations and she agreed that was a fine goal. I feel like I have had much conflict and disappointment in the past month. So, lately I've been saying, "God, make me an instrument of thy peace."

Marianne Williamson says that we receive miracles because we are open to them and know we deserve them.

I suggest taking an online course or trying to read A Course in Miracles yourself. It can be challenging to understand alone

Creating an Altar

An altar in life, alters our life.

Swami Tejomayananda

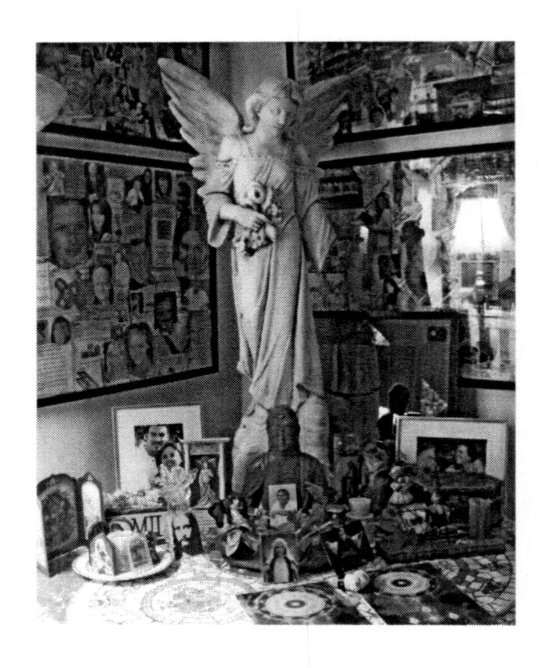

I have an altar in my bedroom that contains symbols of things I love or that have good energy. On my altar right now I have angels, divine figures, a picture of my husband, a sign that says "family," and a collage of my teachers. I also have incense.

It's wonderful to have a sacred area of your room where you can pray, meditate, or just raise your vibration by looking at the altar. If this idea appeals to you, you can make an altar somewhere in your house by using a small table, cloth, pictures or little statues of things you love.

While reading Shakti Gawain's book, *Creative Visualization*, I came upon a sentence where she suggests creating a personal sanctuary *within* yourself. She explains how to imagine that within yourself, you have a beach or ocean or a sacred space you can visit anytime. It's a space of safety and tranquility. It seemed like a good place to go to when you are doing radiation, CAT scans or chemo. An inner altar is beautiful.

So whether you make an altar within or without, remember that by using your imagination and surrounding yourself with peaceful images of things you love, it's another way of coming home to Source.

Taking Things Lightly

There's only enlightenment in the moment. Do you believe a stressful thought? Then you're confused. Do you realize that the thought isn't true? Then you're enlightened to it.

Byron Katie

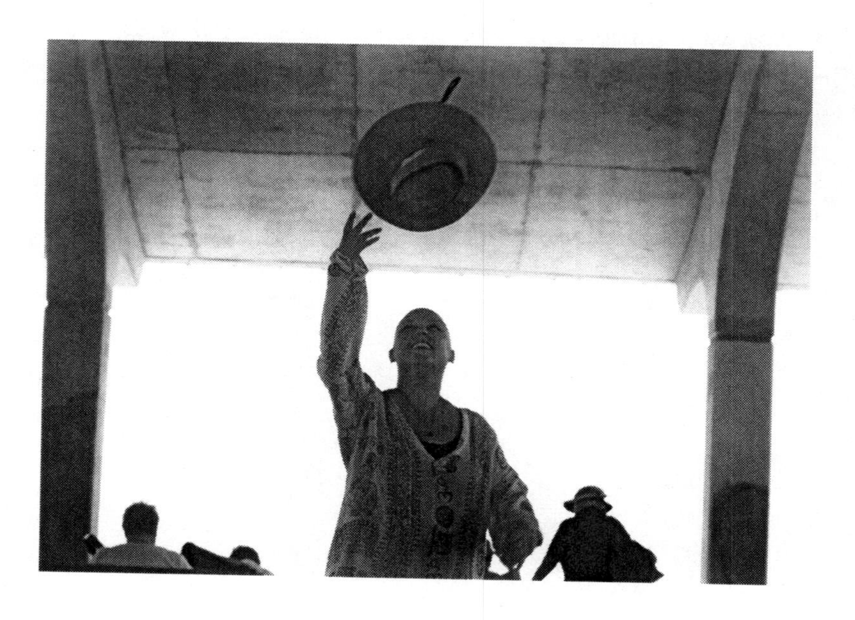

Dr. David Hawkins says that enlightenment is the recognition that one's reality is the light of the self. To me, the process of becoming enlightened means lightening up in the different areas of your life, letting go of attachments, ego, limiting beliefs, and lower vibrations so what is left is love. In her book *Frequency*, Penny Peirce writes, "When intense energy flows through a transparent person, it produces a feeling of heightened divinity, enthusiasm, and light."

The idea of Enlightenment also makes me think of having great trust and a sense of surrender. Doreen Virtue reminds us that straining stems from fear and a lack of trust.

Knock, And He'll open the door
Vanish, And He'll make you shine like the sun
Fall, And He'll raise you to the heavens
Become nothing, And He'll turn you into everything.

RUMI

Trust comes from the root chakra which connects us to Source. A baby just trusts and receives, knowing that he is worthy. He is completely in the moment. When did we lose that seemingly simple ability?

Christopher Dilts once told me that Saint Paul said, "I die daily." I take this to mean that each day he becomes closer to God's will, not his own. When you let go more and more of your old identity while on the Spiritual path, this can feel like a physical death.

Bradley Hess, Director of "Intuitive Energy," helps people return to their Spirit energy by helping them clean it up. He helps them to recognize and release energy that isn't theirs, like limiting beliefs. They clean the junk out of their energy bodies so they can heal themselves and consciously see what they are creating. Brad says it is impossible to discern this on a mental/body level and its only on the energetic level of your Spirit that you can know these things. He says this process is not about learning and developing skills, it's about uncovering parts of ourselves that were buried. He says he helps people ask the question,

"Can I own my own space so I can have the freedom to be who I am?" To me, this is a great way to lighten up and just be. Deepak Chopra describes this when he says, *"It just needs to sink in that letting go is the path to everything."*

In *Angels Are Talking*, Michelle Whitedove says that enlightenment is a state of being where you've mastered unconditional love and grace every day, while in your physical body. Here you come from a place of love no matter what is said or done because you see the intent and lessons behind other people's actions and you don't take anything personally.

I guess one way to lighten up is to look at all the things that push your buttons and try to find humor in them. You will feel much lighter if you can poke humor with yourself. Deepak Chopra counsels, "The crucial times to let go are when you feel the strongest urge not to."

In *Energy Anatomy* Carolyn Myss says that to heal you need to accommodate your energetic system by being able to unplug your circuits. Otherwise, we finance our traumas and limiting beliefs with our cell tissue. This is easier said than done because we have grown comfortable with our inherited beliefs and experiences. When we lighten up we need to be able to forgive past trauma, shed old limiting beliefs, reclaim our own authority, and develop healthy energetic power management skills.

Also, Carolyn Myss points out that mystics can manifest thought into form instantaneously because they aren't plugged into tribal systems. Maybe this is why they say you need to become an empty vessel to channel Spirit. She suggests that we move past our personal agendas and become receptive to guidance that prepares us to take on tasks that serve the greater good.

Louise Hay points out that most good teachers are continually working to release even more, to remove even deeper layers of limitation. She says, "If you think of the hardest thing for you to do and how much you resist it, then you're looking at your greatest lesson at the moment." She encourages us to say to ourselves, "I am willing to change and release all resistance," while looking in the mirror. What is your next challenge to let go of?

Gary Craig (considered the founder of EFT) invented a procedure he calls the Personal Peace Procedure. He suggests making a list of every bothersome specific event from your past and every unwanted emotional response and apply the basic Recipe for tapping to them, one at a time until they do not have a negative impact. At times I have asked life coaching clients to make a similar list so we could work through those issues by talking them through, but I also like the idea of your being able to tap through them, possibly resolving them more quickly. I have not yet learned or tried tapping so I can't attest to its benefits but it sounds like a promising tool and it could not hurt to try it.

The idea is to face your blocks and fears so that you free your energy and can vibrate at a much higher level, choosing love over fear.

Your Spirit Guides

The kingdom of heaven is within.

Joseph Campbell

When you're in the middle of a chaotic experience such as cancer, you probably are hungry for guidance. Saints and avatars are at your disposal, as are people you admire who have passed away. For example, you can pray to Jesus if you are Christian and want to adopt the qualities of mercy or perseverance. If you're Jewish you can pray to the Shekhinah for compassion and faith.

If you're not religious, you can meditate on role models that you admire (even if they are deceased). So, for example, I might meditate on Gandhi for inner conviction and courage or Mother Teresa for unconditional love. If you are in a situation where you need these qualities, you can meditate and ask Mother Teresa, "What would *you* do?" and then just allow the answer to come, without judging it. This can be helpful at a time where you're too identified with a problem of situation and you need to reach for a higher vibration or context.

Another way to get guidance is to go within, to your Higher Self or even to a Spirit guide, like a power animal. When I was in graduate school, I took a class in shamanism at a Goddess Center. They taught us to journey into a deeper level of consciousness to the sound of drumming and then to ask an inner power animal questions, in order to gain new Spiritual wisdom on our physical reality. Whether you connect with your Higher Self, a saint, avatar, teacher or power animal, if the message resonates with you, you will know.

Ted Andrews describes the planes of existence from lower to highest: etheric-nature spirits and elementals, astral-angels and great devas, mental-archangels, intuitive-avatars, monadic-great planetary spirits, and divine-god and goddess. Andrews says it requires only ten minutes a day of meditation to bring more energy and spirit perception into manifestation. He says if you persist for a year it will lead to true clairvoyance.

Andrews suggests that its helpful to eat high vibrational foods, to fast sometimes, to cleanse your aura with salt baths, to drink a lot of water, and that you can burn incense to assist spirit perception. He mentions a number of scents, saying that wisteria (my favorite flower) is one of the scents that can bring you close to guides who promote create inspiration and assist in developing healing energy. He suggests a variety of meditations throughout his book that you can try to foster contact with your spirit guides. He suggests writing down your experiences and any messages you get in your journal.

The 7 Spiritual Gifts of Cancer

When you invoke Heaven, Heaven comes.

CAROLYN MYSS

I believe that you can receive gifts and lessons from most experiences but sometimes you need to look for them. Here are seven of mine:

1. I learned to better balance and be aware of the different parts of myself

2. I became much more clear about my mission and legacy

3. I felt closer to Spirit and to my Higher self than ever before

4. I learned to improve my self-care

5. I tried to look at my karma and how I could love more

6. I became more compassionate as a healer with how tough it is to make changes as a patient

7. I learned that our bodies are our Temple but we are Spirits in physical bodies

When you are toward the end of your journey (or possibly during it) take some time to write about the spiritual gifts that you received, that you might never have received without this cancer experience. Can you find at least 7?

An Initiation into Higher Consciousness

Will you make the non-physical world your authority over the physical?

Carolyn Myss

In writing this book and going through this cancer journey, I already realized that it was an initiation experience and a raising of consciousness. Then I read Michael Mirdad's book, *You're Not Going Crazy . . . You're Just Waking Up!* In it he discusses 5 stages of spiritual transformation where your soul shakes things up in order for you to question your reality. He says that your ego-based life gets dismantled so you can live with your foundation in Spirit. He says that this process often starts when something in your life is stagnant or stuck too long and its ready for a change. He says this is your soul's way of initiating "tough love" and getting a message across that you are ignoring. Most of these are opportunities to understand and experience unconditional love, which Mirdad qualifies as the ability to love not only all of people but all conditions. He says these trials often come in the form of a health crisis, near death experience, or accident. They can also be personal losses or a relationship crisis. He says the stage of emptiness makes us feel as though we're being crucified because our old self is dying and making room for our new self to be born.

The excitement of getting closer to Spirit is not to be minimized. Dr. David Hawkins wrote,

"At first, spiritual purification seems difficult, but eventually, it becomes natural. To consistently choose love, peace, or forgiveness leads one out of the house of mirrors. The joy of God is so exquisite that any sacrifice is worth the effort and seeming pain."

Wake Up Calls

Never lose a holy curiosity.

Albert Einstein

We often feel torn between whether our wake-up calls are predestined or whether it's our job to learn how to balance and solve things as they occur. Maybe it's a little of both. There's an old parable that expresses this paradox:

THE FLOOD

The river is overflowing, the dam is breaking, and an old man is sitting on the porch of his house watching the water rise. He's singing hymns. Along come some members of the national guard in a 4-wheel drive truck. The stop when they see the man. "Come on!" they yell. "The dam is going to break and you will drown." "Nope," answered the man. I'm praying to God and God will provide for me."

The water keeps rising and soon the man is sitting on the porch railing. Along come some more national guardsmen in a motor boat. "Come on!" they yell. "The dam is breaking and all of this is going to be washed away." "Nope," answered the man. I am praying to God and God will provide for me."

The water keeps rising and soon the man is sitting on the roof. A helicopter flies over, stops, and comes back and hovers over him. A ladder is lowered from the helicopter. "Come on!" yells someone from the helicopter. "The dam broke and a wall of water is coming this way!" "Nope," answered the man. I am praying to God and God will provide for me."

Well, the water rolled over the house and this man was swept away and drowned. He soon found himself standing before the Pearly Gates. He asked to see God and was conducted into His presence.

"God," the man said, "I don't understand. I prayed to you and prayed to you and still you let me drown."

"I LET YOU DROWN?" thundered the voice of God. "MY CHILD, I SENT YOU A CAR, A BOAT, AND A HELICOPTER AND EACH TIME YOU TURNED THEM AWAY. WHAT ELSE DID YOU WANT ME TO DO FOR YOU?"

* * *

As applied to our situation, I take this to mean that even if we elected cancer and even if it derives from a divine reason, it's still our job to take this opportunity to heal ourselves. This may mean doing an inventory of body, mind, emotions, and Spirit to see where we need more balance, love, or attention. When we do meet at the pearly gates and do our Life Review, we want to know we did our best to evolve and that we've learned to love ourselves and each other. Consider this book your boat. You are not alone. The tides are rising and we are paddling together against the mass consciousness of fear. Are you in or out?

Near Death Experiences

Until you experience death as a gift,
your work is not done.

Byron Katie

Often when you go through a life-changing experience like cancer, you are faced with life and death issues and with metaphysical and Spiritual questions about the afterlife.

When I was in graduate school in Media, PA, I used to go to Borders to attend book signings and lectures. One time I was browsing the book aisles and sat down in a lecture by the authors Lundahl & Widdison who wrote a book called *The Eternal Journey.* They had interviewed many people who had near death experiences and had found many common themes. I found it fascinating and bought the book. One story I remember was about a man they called DeLynn who had died in an operation and discovered that he had chosen to have cystic fibrosis before being incarnated. He had always hated his disease and wished he hadn't had it. One day DeLynn physically died and in that afterlife state, recalled a scene in a room with an instructor who was saying we can learn lessons on earth slowly with certain experiences or quickly through pain and disease. He wrote Cystic Fibrosis on the board and asked for volunteers. DeLynn remembered raising his hand to accept the challenge, and then he never felt like a victim of his disease again. He knew he couldn't control the deterioration of his physical body but he could control how he handled his illness, both emotionally and psychologically. Once revived, he taught others about their illness. So, sometimes if we know our soul's purpose in our trials and tribulations we can better embrace them with love.

It turns out that 35% of all people who have temporarily died have an NDE—a near death experience. A Gallop poll in 1981 reported that 8 million adults in the US have had a near death experience. In 1990 it was over 22 million—or 1 out of 11 people.

Many people who had near death experiences reported commonalities like a heightened spiritual awareness, they feared death less, believed in an afterlife, mentioned a Life Review and the importance of Love. Many said their near death experience was the most important event in shaping their lives, goals, and activities.

Some people who have had near death experiences report that we choose our whole earth life, including our family and difficulties, and these choices help us progress to a higher level. They said we select our mission and positions for life on earth in order to further our spiritual growth. Many NDEers report having a mission on earth to fulfill that they needed to complete and it usually had to do with helping others.

Sometimes it takes a negative experience to develop our Spirits. Perhaps our spirit is anxious to accept an illness or accident in order to better itself. There is a reason for whatever problems an individual faces. Adversity has a purpose and it isn't punishment. It helps us grow, develop, accomplish our mission and teaches compassion and tolerance.

Many who have had a NDE described it in a similar manner: as a state of Heaven, full of peace and light where things and people glowed from the inside. There were often beautiful gardens (with 3 colors of Wisteria one NDEer described) and choirs of angels singing. People often met deceased relatives and friends from the other side when they first arrived. They even saw huge libraries there because knowledge was important. Gaining knowledge was one way for the spirit to progress in its evolution. You could continue your education for the Higher spheres and help others.

Many people spoke about having a Life Review, which reminded me of Meryl Streep's character in the movie, *Defending Your Life.* A life review is usually described as a 3D movie of your whole life where you get to experience not so much the events of your life, but how you made everyone feel during those events. Interestingly, one NDEer reported that in his Life Review his accomplishments meant nothing: only the small ways he treated others were what seemed most important.

In her book, *Angels are Talking*, psychic Michelle Whitedove says that we go to a Hall of Records when we cross over (this reminded me of Ellis Island) and we review our past lives and learn from our earth experiences. She says that when we reincarnate we get to choose from 2-3 possible lives and we are counseled in this choice by an angel. We have karma and spiritual contracts that need to be fulfilled through mutual agreements with other souls.

Dr. David Hawkins wrote, "Consciousness research confirms that all persons are born under the most optimal conditions for spiritual evolution, no matter what the appearance seems to be. You don't get born without your approval."

Most of these healers say that there are no masks in Heaven so everyone can read each other's thoughts and feelings. People tended to want to speak with others who are at similar levels of light.

I picked up a book on our road trip at a gas station. It was called, *To Heaven and Back: A Doctor's Extraordinary Account of Her Death, Heaven, Angels and Life Again*, by Mary Neal. She was a spine surgeon who was kayaking while on vacation in South America with her husband. She got pinned under the water and drowned. She died and went to heaven and later returned to her body with shattered legs and severe pulmonary problems. She was hospitalized for over a month and was wheelchair bound, yet she considers her accident one of the greatest gifts she ever received. She feels her return to earth was meant to allow her to tell her story to others and to help them find their way back to God.

Not having had an NDE myself, I can't attest to these stories or reports from personal experience. But it was interesting to read about about NDEs and intriguing that so many people reported similar experiences.

The most important thing I learned is that one way or another, it seems we choose our earth challenges so that we can grow, and we are here to learn to love more.

I also thought it was interesting that sometimes confronting death brings out new spiritual gifts and initiations into the Spirit world. I remembered that shamans or healers in other societies often had near death or dismemberment experiences that initiated them into the role of healer. In *Cell-Level Healing*, author Joyce Hawkes explains that a key aspect of training for indigenous healers is facing death. The intent is to conquer fear and be able to walk between physical and spiritual realities. She describes how a healer from Bali might be taken to a temple on an oceanside plot of land only accessible during low tide. The initiates stay there overnight with no food or water, and cobras often emerge from their dens to investigate the intruder. These initiates survive by sitting still in meditation, with no fear.

Carolyn Myss points out that in the Bible, Lazarus was in the tomb before he was resurrected and that some part of us needs to die before a new reality can awaken in us.

In *Your Soul's Plan* by Robert Schwartz, we are told that the majority of life challenges are selected before incarnation, especially our more profound challenges. Schwartz says our lessons become more deeply instilled when we concretize them on the physical plane. The book gives many examples but one that struck me was a homosexual man with AIDS who had been shamed by his family. His choice of nonconformity in this lifetime resulted in his family withdrawing their love, and his lesson was to give himself unconditional love, even if others didn't. His choice to experience judgment and non-conformity led to unconditional love of the self. Similarly, a choice to be very ill and unhealthy could lead someone to value and nurture their body and health afterwards. What lessons might your soul be pressing you to learn with this experience with cancer?

Maybe we can't compare our cancer scare with death to actually dying, but we are confronting fear and the other side more than many people do in their day-to-day life, and I believe this can also be a spiritual initiation of sorts, should we choose to wake up to it.

My friend Bradley Hess, whom I met during graduate school, had a similar occurrence, even though he never physically died. He was at the time an engineer at Bell Labs—a good job that he found fascinating. One day he was starting up his motorcycle, and as he was holding onto it, it surged forward and smashed into a tree. Brad was knocked out and he could feel his Spirit floating 30 feet above his body, and he could see everything below him. He saw his friends in the parking lot pointing and laughing until they realized he was really hurt. His first thought was, "I always swore there was nothing beyond death but I was wrong." He realized that we are a spirit in a physical body and he felt free, wonderful, and peaceful. He realized he was only using 10% of himself in his current job and went to study at Berkeley Psychic Institute. He later started his own center in Pennsylvania, teaching people to understand what they were creating as a Spirit and how to bring that Spiritual energy into our bodies.

Most people who lift the veil temporarily between Heaven and earth are forever changed. As it says in Psalms 23:4, "Yea, though I walk through the valley of the shadow of death, I will fear no evil, for thou art with me." If you gain this type of inner knowing, you have found something eternally lasting.

In Dying to Be Me, the author describes her cancer and how she physically died before returning to her body. After her NDE she had a total remission of her cancer that even the doctors felt was miraculous. Moorjani felt that her prior fear and limiting beliefs fed her cancer, but when she experienced her infinite soul as love on the other side, cancer couldn't exist in that transcendent state. She noticed she had been harsh to herself and couldn't express her full truth prior to having her near death experience. She learned to allow for all possibilities, to surrender, and to trust the wisdom of her Infinite self. She feels that her healing was a result of a spiritual shift in consciousness. She says, "If we get in touch with that infinite place within where we are whole, cancer can't remain."

It was interesting to me that Moorjani reports that for years after being diagnosed with cancer she was vegan, did hypnotherapy, yoga, prayer, mantras, mediation and Chinese herbs but she feels it did not work to heal her because of her beliefs and emotions, especially regarding herself. After her near death experience Moorjani eats what she wants to. She will enjoy chocolate or champagne from time to time and she makes sure that she enjoys her life. She feels that it is more important to be happy than anything else. And if she chooses to eat healthy foods only, then she does so out of love for herself rather than out of fear and misery.

The most common theme of many NDEs is the remembrance that we are love and that we come here to earth to learn lessons about unconditional love, joy, and service. According to Schwartz in *Your Soul's Plan*, what looks like suffering on the physical plane is temporary but the wisdom we gain is eternal.

Your Personal Experience With Death

She holds nothing back from life;
therefore she is ready for death.

Byron Katie

Sometimes it's only when a loved one dies or when we are confronted with a near death experience or illness that we let ourselves think about death. Even though many times our death is uncontrollable, contemplating our death ahead of time can help us to make meaning of it and consider how we would like that transition to be for us.

So, start by getting into a relaxed loving state (instead of the fearful state that death normally evokes) and ask yourself, *"What does death mean to me?"* Do you believe in heaven and that your spirit will live on? What might be the greatest thing about dying? What is the most challenging thing to you? Journal about this for a while.

Okay, assuming you have a context for reflecting on death, how might you prepare for this transition, should it happen? Are there certain practicalities that you have put in place? For example, do you have life insurance? Did you create a will? We did one on www.legalzoom.com for $25 and it was very quick. Did you leave letters or a video or albums for your loved ones? What would you like at your funeral or memorial? Where and how would you like to be buried, or cremated? Who would you want there? Take a moment to write out these particulars. You can even start a file of your wishes for this transition and appoint someone to be in charge of it. Perhaps you want to make sure everyone knows how much you love them. As Emily Dickinson once wrote, "Unable are the Loved to die, for love is immortality."

I like the saying, "Plan for the best but prepare for the worst." Let's plan that we will all beat cancer and live long happy, healthy lives, but we can prepare for an eventual transition. Use this section to do this for yourself and your loved ones.

There is also a book I found called, *What My Family Should Know*, where you can record all important information about your life insurance, bank accounts, financial accounts, safe deposit box information, real estate, social security information, business, professional advisors, your recommendations, etcetera. I will put a link to this product in my Resource section.

Leaving Behind a Legacy

Each of us needs all the positive legacies we can get;
if you fail to share yours, someone is going to be one legacy short.

DANIEL TAYLOR

No one is saying that you are going to die, but having a medical scare makes you think about death, right? It did for me. I wanted to leave a legacy, which is something that people remember you by and your way of contributing to the world. According to Daniel Taylor in *Creating a Spiritual Legacy*, a spiritual legacy passes along your wisdom.

Whether we think it consciously or not, we all have a legacy. It is the sum total of our deeds, relationships, work, laughter, and achievements. I would leave behind a husband, two children, family, friends, patients, students, and a life of 42 years. Still, when I got my diagnosis I understood that I wanted to publish 22 books as a legacy project, in order to put my messages into the world.

Your legacy can be something used at your funeral, read by your great grandkids to get to know you long after you're gone, or, if you're still here in twenty years it can be a tool to share your story. Either way it's a satisfying transitional gift that will remain in our transitory physical world long after your physical body is gone.

I was surprised that more hospitals don't offer Legacy programs for patients who are, or may be, terminally ill. For example, Sloan Kettering Hospital in New York runs a program called Visible Ink, where you can write your story with volunteer editors. Do contact your hospital social worker to inquire what resources might be available in your area.

You don't need to feel that you have to do something so ambitious as writing a book (while you're already tired and struggling with your illness) but you may feel inspired to do something. Some people blog, journal, create a memory book, write an autobiography, create a video, organize home movies, write letters to loved ones, start a charity, create a spiritual will or create art work.

I think it can be comforting to leave behind something of beauty that houses your experience and is lasting. In "Playing Among the Dead" (my doctoral dissertation) I described how Holocaust survivors and their families found ingenious ways to leave creative legacies, both during their Holocaust experience and afterwards, and how this was healing.

If you have ever seen the films *My Life* or *Stepmom*, they are great examples of leaving a legacy. In *My Life* the main character creates home movies for his wife and child. In *Stepmom* the mom who is dying creates a beautiful handmade cape for her son. In *My Life Without Me* the main character is dying and records tapes for her daughters every birthday, as well as messages for other family members. This film is worth watching.

What might you like to do?

I will give you an example of a *Spiritual Will* below and then provide you with a list of related legacy resources to get you started.

Here is my *Spiritual Will—15 Life Lessons I Learned:*

1. Be creative and bring your heart and soul to all you do.

2. Live from your center and Love who you are.

3. Love as much as you can- both yourself and others.

4. Take time to connect to your soul and Higher Self. This is the eternal essence of who you are.

5. Notice when you are judging or in pain and try to raise your vibration to love and acceptance (as much as you are able to).

6. Try and enjoy and praise your life every day, even if you begin with 30 minutes.

7. Reflect on why you are here and the lessons that you are learning.

8. Appreciate the good and beauty in yourself and others, even when you are at your worst, or they are.

9. Try and leave part of your Light behind in your legacies—creative acts with the world in mind.

10. Learn to trust your inner wisdom and find great Spiritual teachers too.

11. Remember that we are all One and that we need to respect and learn from both our differences and our similarities.

12. Challenges come bearing gifts, so look for them and grow.

13. Try and choose love instead of fear. Learn to catch the difference in each moment.

14. Hug people and say, "I Love You" a lot.

15. Remember that you're not alone. You have yourself, your angels and your earth angels. Try and learn from everyone, especially yourself!

You can number and write your own 15 Spiritual lessons. Or, write a poem or short story about your cancer experience, organize home movies, write letters, blog, journal or make a video to your loved ones. If you need help, you can give someone your pictures and pay them to make a scrapbook for you or create a video of your story. I've listed some resources below for help.

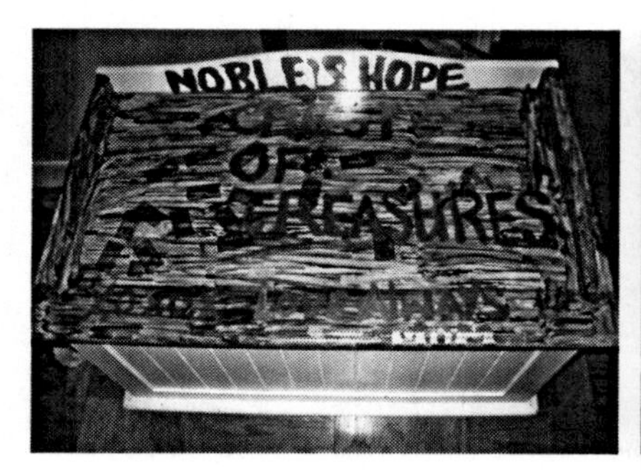

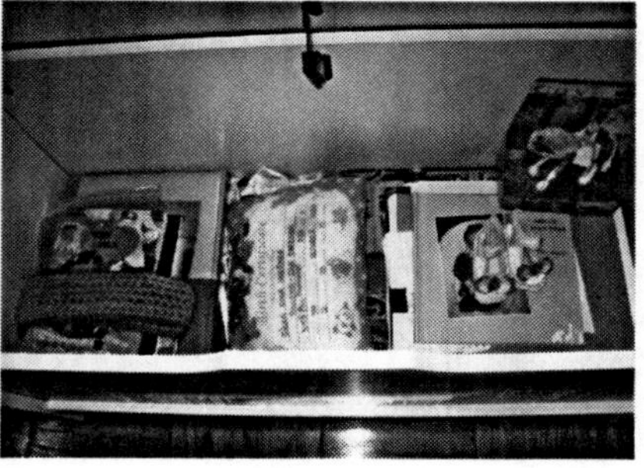

I decided to make Hope Chests for my 2 year old daughter Sera and my 4 year old son Noble. Then I was inspired to make one for my husband too. This led to memory boxes that I decoupaged for each of my parents. I included personalized photo albums, a letter, special cards, home movies or sentimental items (like my daughters hospital outfit) and the 9 books I had published so far. I don't know how I made the time to do this while I was recovering and working but it gave me peace of mind to know that if I died, I was leaving some important messages behind for them. It was also fun to use my heart and creativity this way. You can consider whether a project like this would be fun for you too. Even though I believe that I will live a long life, it makes me smile thinking about my kids opening these chests when they are 40 years old!

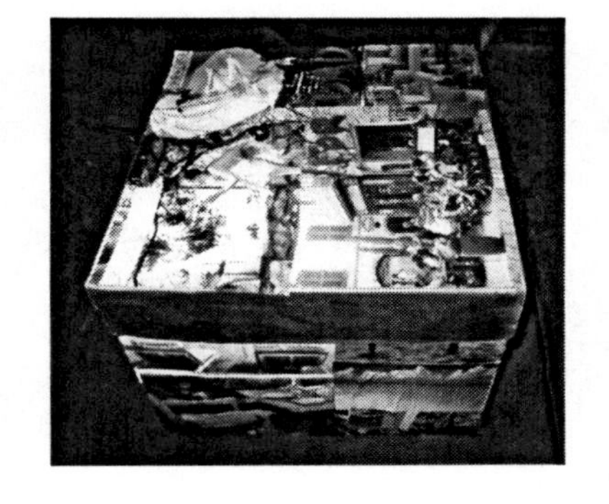

YOUR LEGACY RESOURCE LIST

Association of Personal Historians (www.personalhistorians.org) You can hire experts to help you write a book or videotape your story here.

Story Corps (storycorps.org) Their mission is to provide Americans of all backgrounds and beliefs with the opportunity to record, share, and preserve the stories of our lives. They sometimes come to your area for free or they have a do it yourself kit.

Everyone Has a Story (everyonehasastory.net) Here's one example of a company that will film your legacy. I did not try them and there are probably many others in your area if you don't want to do it yourself.

Patient Voices (www.patientvoices.org.uk) A website of patient stories

Program in Narrative Medicine (www.narrativemedicine.org) A program at Columbia University. Director Dr. Rita Charon.

SOME SCRAPBOOKING RESOURCES

Scrapbooking for You (scrapbookingforyou.tripod.com/index-a.html) People who will scrapbook for you.

Treasured Memories & More
(treasuredmemoriesmor.tripod.com/id3.html) Scrapbooking for you.

Heritage Makers (www.heritagemakers.com)

Snapfish (www.snapfish.com)

Wholeness, Completion & Cycles

The kingdom of Heaven will become one with the kingdom of Earth and the Lord will reign forever and ever.

Revelations 11:5

I finished my last radiation treatment in October, 2012, so it feels like a large part of this journey is over and maybe I can put cancer behind me soon. It seems like an appropriate time for an ending because the leaves are changing and the earth is sending me messages that fall is here. Autumn symbolizes letting go, letting Spirit take over, and balancing light and dark within. To Christians who observe the liturgical year, autumn is actually the beginning of the cycle so this feels like both an ending and a beginning, like coming full circle, and finding my way home again.

My husband and I wanted to have a celebratory mini-break, so grandma watched our kids and we took a long weekend road trip to Niagara Falls. We drove 7 hours to a bed and breakfast in Fredonia, NY to sleep over.

The next day we drove to Niagara Falls and rode the Maid of the Mist boat on the U.S. side. It was so misty out, just like on my first date with my husband. I looked up the symbolism of mist and it said that it is similar to a veil, it is the transition to seeing clearly and resolving your current dilemma. It is divinity letting us know that what we are looking for is in our sight: a prelude to an important manifestation.

Here are the powerful falls:

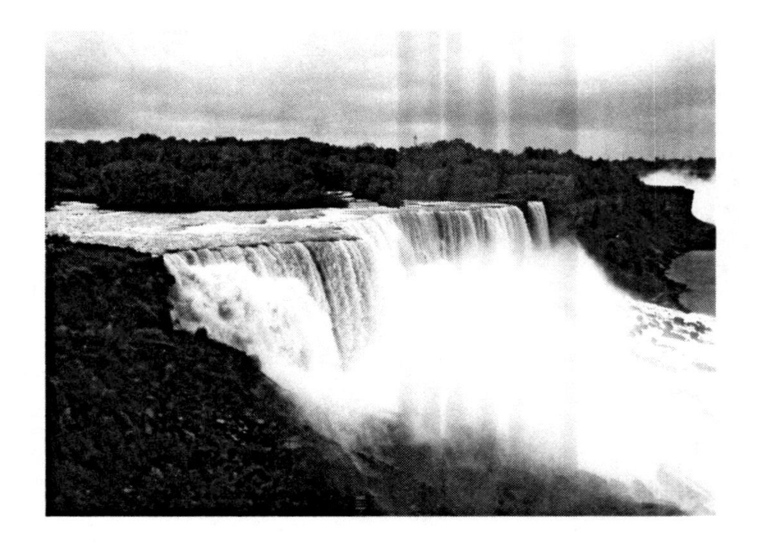

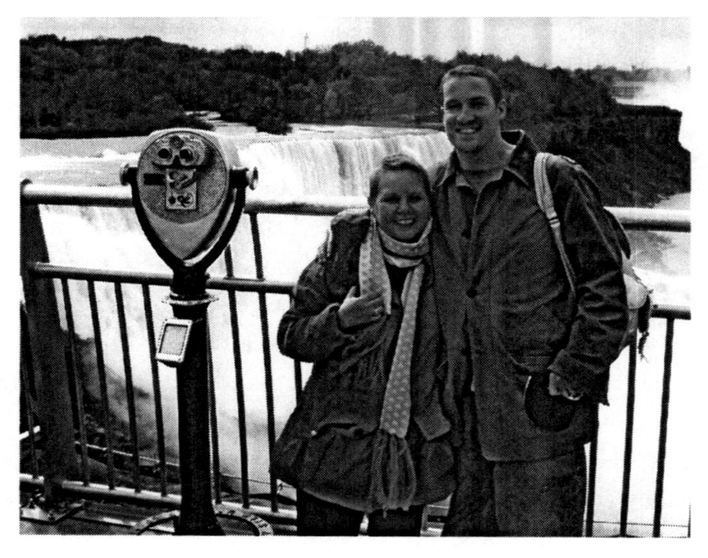

HERE IS ME WITH MY HONEY

Then we drove to the Canadian side of the falls and rode the Ferris wheel at night. The falls were lit up in many colors which reminded me of the night that we got engaged. My husband proposed on the beach in Coney Island and afterwards we rode the Ferris wheel and looked out on our life ahead. This time I feel like we looked out on all we'd been through together in the past year and now it was finally time to move past it.

On the way home we stopped at a Denny's and they asked us to donate $1 for cancer, which we did. I felt surrounded by support there, seeing all the cookies/donations that people had contributed:

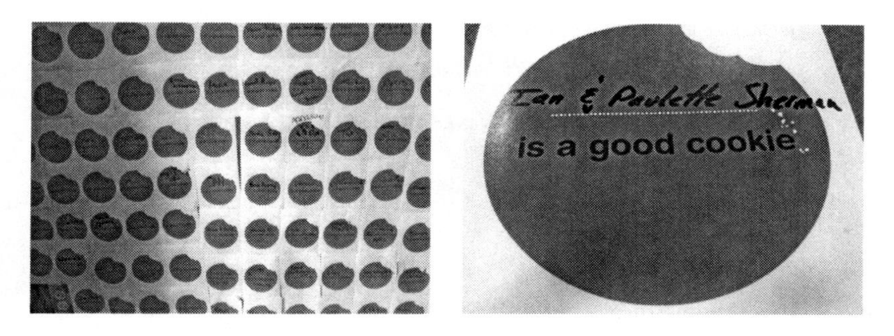

DENNY'S CANCER DONATION PROGRAM CALLED COOKIES FOR KIDS' CANCER.

I got my period too (and even though that isn't fun), for me it was a sign that my early menopause wasn't permanent and that my body was reverting to normal, even at 42 years old. I had been without my period for 6 months during treatment so it felt good to return to normal, even though we did not want more kids and were told not to get pregnant for at least two years anyway.

November ended with Thanksgiving. I had a lot to be grateful for. I received so much help and love during my journey and hopefully I would be fine. I realize others aren't so lucky and many have lost loved ones to cancer. But I hope I receive lots of emails from those of you who survive, thrive and have even more love than ever before!

Afterword

Do not go where the path may lead.
Go instead where there is no path
and leave a trail.

Ralph Waldo Emerson

Looking back, this cancer path was my Alice in Wonderland or Wizard of Oz journey through cancer. I fell through a rabbit hole and spent time on a deeper level enlarging my views, looking at my subconscious fears and issues, examining symbolism, healing energy and parts of myself that the eye doesn't see.

It helped to scribble out a tome of a book while I was in treatment so I could process and absorb everything. While I was walking the beach, I got a revelation that it was meant to be a 4-volume series called *The Cancer Path* that would embrace other women with cancer at different points along their journey.

My first book, Volume 1 was called *My Quick Guide Through Breast Cancer: Diagnosis, Surgery, Chemo & Radiation*. This was that first cancer gift book that would connect you to someone else who had this experience and provide you with an overview and some practical tips about how to get through surgery, chemo, or radiation. Some women prefer just to get those tips, get through their conventional hospital treatment and put cancer behind them, and stop there. This first book can guide them through this first cancer path.

Volume 2 is the book you are now holding: *The Cancer Path: A Spiritual Journey Through Healing, Wholeness & Love.* This book is from my heart and it approaches cancer as a spiritual initiation, on a level deeper. It allows you to heal your cancer from the inside-out by giving you tools to address your mind, body, emotions, and Spirit as you go through your traditional hospital treatment. If you are like me, you may not want to be a passive recipient of healing. You may want to take action and create a year of treatment that leads to greater wholeness and health on all levels. I read over 60 books so that I could address these four levels of healing for you, as well as explore many discrepant issues such as your diet, how your immune system affects cancer, whether emotions, thoughts and stress affect cancer etcetera. So this book is for the cancer patient who wants to do serious inner work and learn spiritual lessons along this path so she will become a Spiritual initiate.

Volume 3 in this series is called *My Date With Cancer: 21 Spiritual Lessons.* It is a gift book that explores 21 of the Spiritual lessons from book #2 without the more intensive research and exercises. It's a short gift book with color pictures and brief spiritual lessons that a cancer patient can flip through while in the hospital. It's intended to provide love and hope and point out some things that will help patients grow and be positive while on their cancer journey.

Volume 4- *Create Your Own Cancer Path Workbook* is a workbook that helps cancer patients keep track of their personal experience and story. It is a journal/workbook with ideas, springboards and exercises so that they can remember how they got through chemotherapy, people who inspired them, what lessons they learned, and so on. In the end, people can use this workbook as a template for writing and publishing their own story, if they wish. This can be a legacy for their children, grand-children, and great-grand children to learn from their story. I found writing to be very therapeutic. Research shows that there are many benefits to cancer patients from journaling and leaving a legacy behind.

Now that my cancer treatment is finally over (and hopefully my cancer is gone forever) I hope I've helped others with my experience. I hope to continue this growth path well beyond my cancer but sometimes I worry that I will revert to my comfort zone.

Michael Mirdad writes, "All initiations, no matter how simple or profound, must be integrated into your life and become part of who you are."

I started vegetable juicing at home and drinking alkalized water. I use mostly Stevia instead of sugar and eliminated most bread and flour. I am making progress in changing my dietary ways.

I realized that I was good at coping with pain and reducing it through mental, spiritual, and coping strategies, as I have helped people to do for years. What was more challenging for me, was to switch my focus from mastering pain to embracing love in every moment. After treatment I needed to use all aspects of myself to choose health, indefinitely.

If I'm honest, losing my hair, and braving many physical symptoms and scary procedures for a year seemed in some ways easier than facing a lifetime of healthy eating, choosing loving thoughts, meditation, colonics, praying, and exercise on a daily basis, in addition to all my regular responsibilities! There, I've said it, and as embarrassing as it is, maybe you feel that way sometimes too.

But what we focus on expands. We can recreate ourselves and our cells in each minute with our love. Our doctors too can shift from the "decrease pain and eliminate disease" paradigm to the *increase overall health for quality of life* model.

I believe that medicine is going to merge more with energy medicine, epigenetics, and quantum physics in the future. In Bruce Lipton's book, *The Biology of Belief*, he speaks about his own paradigm shift as a cellular biologist which allowed him to see life in a whole new way when he realized that our cells respond to their environment and to our behavior.

It is important for us to take a holistic view because all four levels of mind, body, emotions and Spirit that we've discussed effect each other. Even scientists and doctors will eventually prove and accept this notion.

For example, the field of Epigenetics explores how environmental signals select, modify, and regulate our gene activity, according to Bruce Lipton. He found that when he adjusted things to create a healthy environment, "sick cells" revived. He points out that single-gene disorders affect less than 2% of the population. Most people have genes that enable a happy, healthy life so it's what we do that also affects them. He says that diabetes, cancer, and heart disorders have complex interactions among multiple genes and environmental factors. Environment, stress, emotion, thinking, and nutrition can modify them without changing their blueprint. Interestingly, these modifications can even be passed on to future generations! Dr. Dean Ornish revealed that by changing the diet and lifestyle of prostate cancer patients for 90 days, he switched the activity of over 500 genes and many of those gene changes inhibited biological processes critical to forming tumors.

Speaking of lifestyle changes, I recently called my oncologist to ask if he would recommend an integrative medicine doctor who would hopefully take my insurance and who would monitor my diet, blood levels, vitamins and minerals, after I finished my chemo. He did not know one and his secretary said none of the patients who'd been through chemotherapy ever asked this. I explained that if the cancer is eliminated and I build back my immune system I could remain cancer-free but if the cancer returns, it will be terminal. So this was an important window for me. I felt that I should focus on building up my immune system, taking supplements and minerals, looking at my blood work, killer-cells and diet, and give my body a lot of care and love. The secretary said they normally saw patients three months after chemotherapy for a general blood test and assumed that patient's immune system would come back on their own.

So I called a number of doctors in NYC listed in the back of Suzanne Somers' book, *Knockout*, on my own. One doctor called back and told me, "Not only do I not take insurance. No one in Manhattan does." So, what's a person to do . . . spend $14,000 for a program like Dr. Gonzalez's or about $4200 a week for Gerson's program in Mexico (on their website they have a home program for $125)? One doctor named Dr. Salerno that I found in Somers' book accepted some out-of-network reimbursement and his secretary would submit billing to your insurance for you. Also the blood work and labs were covered by my insurance so I am going to try and see him. If doctors were more open to this need than an integrative medicine doctor could be on staff at the hospital and insurance would cover it. In Germany, alternative medicine is covered so we have a ways to go here in the United States. Another website for integrative or holistic doctors is: http://holisticmedicine.org/- the American Holistic Medical Association.

If you cannot afford to have a doctor oversee your supplements you can at least do vegetable juicing, drink alkalinized water, exercise, meditate, and have a good doctor monitor your blood work and killer-cells.

Now that cancer may really be gone and the new year is on the horizon, I ask myself, "Was this journey a dream world of my own making; a way to cope and make meaning of a frightful experience? Was it the scientific hospital treatment of chemotherapy and radiation that cured me, or the journey itself that was most healing? Will I continue to see the world in this spiritual light on a regular basis?" I hope so.

And, is it strange to be somewhat positive about having cancer? The other day I got a fortune cookie that said, *"It's better to be an optimist and be proven a fool than to be a pessimist and be proven right."* This seemed like a clue to answering that question! I was hoping to add some light, hope and healing to this previously scary and dark world of cancer.

And as I initially warned, I'm asking more questions than giving answers here. My father read my first draft and asked how this was a self-help book if I could not say that yoga or meditation *would* definitely cure cancer. Ah, if only life were so clear and simple. Isn't it possible that help is on a continuum and it isn't universally absolute?

The truth is, I am the patient *and* the healer, and so are you.

As patient, I feel like this is that moment where Bridget in the movie *Bridget Jones Diary* pauses to consider how many pounds she's lost and how many cigarettes she's still smoking.

I still need to lose 30 pounds, exercise and improve my diet but I did much more self-care than before and my habits *have* improved. Also some shifts were more profound and intangible because they've permeated my world view. And there's no qualification for my renewed connection to Spirit, Higher Self, and my soul's mission, for all of which I am grateful.

And although cancer is hopefully over, my spiritual evolution continues. In *The Path to Love*, Deepak Chopra says, "It is alright to be aware of a distance between vision and reality, because that is what it feels like to be on the path. If you had no gaps to close, you wouldn't need a path."

In this book I've tried to present different sides to multiple questions. Paradox is an opportunity to create greater balance, wholeness and to bridge the Feminine and Masculine, Yin and Yang, mind, body and Spirit, and Eastern and Western medicine.

Doctors may read this foray into angels, auras, and metaphysical healers and perceive it as a joke. But Metaphysics joins science and ancient wisdom, and we will be seeing more partnership between these areas, both within ourselves and in our outer society and healthcare.

I also think that spiritually speaking, the veil between earth and heaven is lifting. Some of us no longer *only* believe what we can see with our eyes or prove in a laboratory setting. We know that the temple is within and that our Spirit is more powerful than our body. Some of us are starting to believe that we are Spirits that change bodies and live on in different forms. Our truth may run deeper than this three-dimensional world and if we are willing to release our fear and be open to love, we may reveal higher frequencies of light in all domains.

I wonder whether my personal healing experience with cancer applies to a larger group. Marianne Williamson says, "Personal transformation can and does have global effects. As we go, so goes the world, for the world is us. The revolution that will save the world is ultimately a personal one." And I guess I believe that too.

Would I have done this healing without cancer? Perhaps I would have just remained with eyes closed and I needed this encounter with darkness to bring on more light.

I'm grateful to have traveled this path and I hope that you too come through it with more light, love, higher consciousness, and strength than ever before, allowing it to soften you and bring that love and compassion to others.

I'm not saying that cancer isn't painful, that life isn't sometimes unfair and that people can't be cruel at the worst times. I have seen that on this journey too. It can also be a ton of work getting through treatment and back to health. It can be even harder moving from fear to love when you are in the middle of a life-threatening illness. It's important to remember that from the perspective of ego and the physical world, most things are a struggle. But from the perspective of Spirit, everything brings a lesson in its right time that can lead to greater peace and wholeness. So, in a way, both are true.

I'm happy to have spent time on this planet and I hope I will continue to be here a long time. Please continue to spread love instead of fear and war because as we have all seen, this lower frequency energy is not good for our bodies, our planet, or our society. And I would love to see us all flourish.

I began this book with a quote from *Conversations with God*, channeled by Neale Donald Walsch, *"God has sent you nothing but angels,"* because at the Spiritual level we can use everything to evolve. Our bodies may be finite but our Spirit is infinite and being that it's part of God, it remains an eternal source of wisdom, love and unity. We just need to learn how to tap into it. And hopefully, this journey will give you a running start.

I wish you many Blessings and much healing on your path, and love, *much* love.

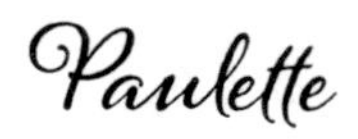

Bibliography

Achterberg, Jeanne & Barbara Dossey. (1994). *Rituals of Healing: Using Imagery for Health and Wellness*. New York: Bantam Books.

Andrews, Ted. (2009). *How to Heal With Color*. MN: Llewellyn Publications.

Andrews, Ted. (1997). *How to Meet and Work with Spirit Guides*. MN: Llewellyn Publications.

Andrews, Ted. (2009). *The Healer's Manual*. MN: Llewellyn Publications.

Baird, James & Nadel, Laurie. (2010). *Happiness Genes*. NJ: New Page Books.

Bolinger, Ty. *Cancer: Step Outside the Box*. TX: Infinity 510 Partners.

Boutenko, Victoria. (2009). *Green Smoothie Revolution*. CA: North Atlantic Books.

Brown, R. (1989). Creativity: What Are We to Measure? In J.A. Glover, R.R Ronning and C.R. Reynolds (Eds.), *Handbook of Creativity* (p.3-32). NY: Plenum.

Brown, Roxanne. (2011). *Chemo: Secrets to Thriving*. IN: NorLights Press.

Byron, Katie. (2007). *A Thousand Names of Joy.* New York: Three Rivers Press.

Calbom, Cherie. (2010). *The Juice Lady's Turbo Diet.* FL: Siloam.

Calbom, Calbom & Mahaffey. (2006). *The Complete Cancer Cleanse.* TN: Thomas Nelson.

Carr, Kris. (2012). *Crazy Sexy Kitchen: 150 Plant-Empowered Recipes to Ignite a Mouthwatering Revolution*. CA: Hay House.

Carr, Kris. (2007). *Crazy, Sexy Cancer Tips.* CT: Skirt Press!

Carr, Kris. (2011). *Crazy, Sexy Diet.* CT: Skirt Press!

Chodron, Pema. (2005). *The Places that Scare You*. Boston: Shambhala.

Chopra, Deepak. (2009). *Reinventing the Body, Resurrecting the Soul.* NY: Three Rivers Press.

Chopra, Deepak. (1996). *The Path to Love.* NY: Harmony.

Chopra, Deepak. (1989). *Quantum Healing.* NY: Bantam Books.

Choquette, Sonia. (2008). *Soul Lessons & Soul Purpose.* CA: Hay House.

Cobb, Brenda. (2002). *The Living Foods Lifestyle.* GE: Living Soul Publishing.

Des Pres, Terrence (1976). *The Survivor: An Anatomy of Life in the Death Camps.* NY: Oxford University Press.

Dossey, Larry. (1996). *Prayer is Good Medicine.* CA: HarperOne.

Dwoskin, Hale. (2003). *The Sedona Method.* AZ: Sedona Press.

Eden, Donna. (2008). *Energy Medicine.* NY: Tarcher/Penguin.

Feinstein, David, Eden, Donna & Craig, G. (2005). *The Promise of Energy Psychology.* NY: Tarcher/Penguin.

Frankl, Viktor. (2006). *Man's Search for Meaning.* NY: Beacon Press.

Gawain, Shakti. (2008). *Creative Visualization.* CA: New World Library.

Geffen, Jeremy. (2000). *The Journey Through Cancer.* NY: Three Rivers Press.

Goleman, Daniel. (2003). *Healing Emotions: Conversations with the Dalai Lama on Mindfulness, Emotions and Health.* London: Shambhala.

Hanson, Rick. (2009). *Buddha's Brain: The Practical Neuroscience of Happiness, Love & Wisdom.* CA: New Harbinger Publications.

Harra, Carmen (2001). *Wholeliness.* CA: Hay House.

Hawkes, Joyce. (2006). *Cell-Level Healing.* NY: Atria Books.

Hawkins, David. (2006). *Transcending the Levels of Consciousness.* AZ: Veritas Publishing.

Hawkins, David. (2009). *Healing and Recovery.* AZ: Veritas Publishing.

Hawkins, David. (2012). *Power Versus Force.* AZ: Veritas Publishing.

Hawkins, David. (2011). *Dissolving the Ego, Realizing the Self.* CA: Hay House.

Hay, Louise. (1991). *The Power is Within You.* CA: Hay House.

Hay, Louise. (1999). *You Can Heal Your Life.* CA: Hay House.

Hay, Louise. (2004). *I Can Do It.* CA: Hay House.

Hay, Louise & Richardson, Cheryl (2011). *You Can Create an Exceptional Life.* CA: Hay House.

Hubbard, Barbara (2001). *Emergence.* VA: Hampton Roads.

Huffington, Ariana. (1994). *The Fourth Instinct.* NY: Simon & Schuster.

Judith, Anodea. (1987). *Wheels of Light*. MN: Llewellyn Publications; 1st edition.

Kamm, Laura. (2006). *Intuitive Wellness*. NY: Atria Books.

Keyes, Raven. (2012). *The Healing Power of Reiki*. MN: Llewellyn Publications.

Kushner, Harold. (1981). *When Bad Things Happen to Good People*. NY: Anchor Books.

Logan, Karen. (1997). *Clean House, Clean Planet*. NY: Pocket Books.

Lapin, Jackie. (2007). *The Art of Conscious Creation*. SC: Elevate.

Lipton, Bruce. (2008). *The Biology of Belief.* CA: Hay House.

Lundahl & Widdison. (1997). *The Eternal Journey*. New York: Warner Books.

MacGregor, Catriona (2010). *Partnering with Nature*. New York: Atria Books.

Mirdad, Michael. (2009). *You're Not Going Crazy, You're Just Waking Up!* WA: Grail Press.

Mirdad, Michael. (2011). *Healing the Heart and Soul*. WA: Grail Press.

Moorjani, Anita. (2012). *Dying To Be Me*. CA: Hay House.

Myss, Carolyn. (1997). *Energy Anatomy*. CO: Sounds True.

Neil, Mary. (2011). *To Heaven and Back: A Doctor's Extraordinary Account of Her Death, Heaven, Angels and Life Again*. CO: Waterbrook Press.

Ovitz, Lori. (2004). *Facing the Mirror with Cancer*. Chicago: Belle Press.

Pierce, Penny. (2009). *Frequency*. New York: Atria Books.

Pressman, Steven. (2002). *The War of Art*. NY: Warner Books.

Schwartz, Robert. (2007). *Your Soul's Plan*. CA: Frog Books.

Selub, Eva. (2009). *The Love Response*. Ballantine Books.

Sherman, Paulette. (2008). *Dating from the Inside Out: How to Use the Law of Attraction in Matters of the Heart*. NY: Atria Books.

Sherman, Paulette. (2013). *My Quick Guide Through Breast Cancer: Diagnosis, Surgery, Chemo & Radiation*. NY: Parachute Jump Publishing.

Sherman, Paulette. (2013). *The Create Your Own Cancer Path Workbook*. NY: Parachute Jump Publishing.

Siegal, Bernie. (1990). *Love, Medicine & Miracles*. NY: William Morrow Paperbacks.

Silberstein, Susan (2009). *Breast Cancer: Is It What You're Eating or What's Eating You?*. PA: Center for Advancement in Cancer Education.

Silva, Jose. (1977). *The Silva Mind Control Method*. New York: Pocket Books.

Somers, Suzanne. (2009). *Knockout: Interviews with Doctors Who Are Curing Cancer*. NY: Three Rivers Press.

Taylor, Daniel. (2011). *Creating a Spiritual Legacy*. NY: Brazos Press.

Walsch, Neale Donald. (2003). *Conversations With God: An Uncommon Dialogue, Book 3*. MA: Hampton Roads Publisher.

White, M. & Epstein, D. (1990). *Narrative Means to Therapeutic Ends*. NY: WW Norton.

Whitedove, Michelle. (2000). *She Talks With Angels*. FL: Whitedove Press.

Whitedove, Michelle. (2002). *The Angels Are Talking*. FL: Whitedove Press.

Other Resources

RELEVANT ARTICLES

Kolata, Gina. "Is There a Link Between Stress and Cancer?," found in the *New York Times*, November 29, 2005.

Xiao-Dong Sun, Xing-E Liu, Dong-Sheng Huang. Curcumin induces apoptosis of triple-negative breast cancer cells by inhibition of EGFR expression. *Mol Med Report*. 2012 Sep 26. Epub 2012 Sep 26.

FILMS

Fierce Grace by Ram Das
City of Angels
One a Minute
Lorenzo's Oil
My Life
Stepmom
Crazy, Sexy Cancer
My Sister's Keeper
Five
Matters of Life and Dating
Living Proof

Why I Wore Lipstick to my Mastectomy
Farrah's Story
Sweet November
A Walk to Remember
My Life Without Me
Life as a House
My Life
Dying Young
Wit
One True Thing
Erin Brockovich
The Bucket List
A Message from Holly
A Little Bit of Heaven
50/50
First Do No Harm
Cancer Conquest
The Cure Is
Now is Good

MOVEMENT

Chakra Balancing DVD—starring Sharon Gannon (Feb 3, 2009).

IMMUNE SYSTEM SELF-HYPNOSIS CD

Order the *Optimal Health: Immune System Enhancement* CD (www.drbereedarby.com).

MEDITATION

Meditation 1: Self Healing (8 CD set) by Bradley Hess. (www.intuitiveenergy.com).

Breathing: The Master Key of Self-Healing by Andrew Weil, MD.

CANCER

Cancer: Discovering Your Healing Power by Louise Hay. An audio CD by Hay House.

A Meditation to Help You Fight Cancer by Bellruth Naparstek. An audio CD.

CHANGE

Change & Transition by Louise Hay (CD).

SELF-ESTEEM

How to Love Yourself by Louise Hay (2005).

ANGER

Anger Releasing by Louise Hay. An audio CD by Hay House.

FEAR

Overcoming Fears by Louise Hay. An audio CD by Hay House.

ANGELS

The Temple of Angelic Healing-Volume 1 by LaUna Huffines. See: www.healingwithlight.org/web/products/index.html

Doreen Virtue's *Manifesting with the Angels*. See www.hayhouse.com.

Christopher Dilts—YouTube angel meditation. See his website: www.askanangel.org

CONNECTING WITH YOUR GUIDES

Channeling: What It Is and How to Do It by Lita De Alberti.

AFFIRMATIONS

Self Esteem Affirmations by Louise Hay (CD).

CHAKRAS

Anodea Judith's DVD: *The Illuminated Chakras* (September 8, 2010).

Carolyn Myss's *Energy Anatomy* DVD.

Chakra Balancing DVD-starring Sharon Gannon (Feb 3, 2009).

LOVE

Becoming Love DVD by Lita DeAlberdi.
See: www.schoolofthelivinglight.co.uk/about-the-school/lita-de-alberdi/ or product page for CDs.

Look on www.theloveresponse.com for *'The Love Response: 10 Minutes to Relax'* audio book or download meditations on breast health.

MANIFESTATION

Attracting Success by Sandra Anne Taylor.

ORACLE DECKS

The Nature-Speak Oracle by Ted Andrews.

Archangel Oracle Cards by Doreen Virtue.

Magical Messages for the Fairies by Doreen Virtue.

Messages from Your Angels by Doreen Virtue.

TAPPING

The Tapping Solution by Nicholas Ortner (thetappingsolution.org).

INTUITION

John Holland's four CD set, *Awakening Your Psychic Strengths*. See www.hayhouse.com.

A COURSE IN MIRACLES

Marianne Williamson's DVD, *Being in Light*. See www.hayhouse.com.

CHANTING

Michelle Newman (www.facebook.com/SingYourSoulSong) She leads Soulsong workshops for women with cancer and is a sound healer who uses her voice and crystal bowls.

PLACES FOR SPIRITUAL CLASSES AND LEARNING–ONLINE OR IN PERSON

Namaste Bookstore (www.namastebookshop.com)

The Open Center (www.opencenter.org)

Omega (www.eomega.org)

Hay House (www.hayhouse.com)

The Learning Annex (www.learningannex.com) online classes are often less than $10

OTHER THINGS

Orange-blue sunglasses for sleep.

Quest brownie flavored bars a dessert or snack alternative. Order on Amazon.

Liquid Splenda, french vanilla flavored (instead of sugar).

Beekley Medical S-Spot for Mammography Skin Stickers.

Mannatech Products—*Glyco Bears*, 1-800-779-0897.

Wolfe Clinic Canada—*Vital Peptide Sachets*, 1-877-359-6950 (for after treatment to raise your immune system).

High Vibe (www.highvibe.com) great site for food products and recipes.

Queasy Pops—3 pops for $10 at www.chemochicks.com.

Life Wave Nanotechnology Patch of Glutathione (www.suzannesomers.com/lifewave).

Coleman Natural (www.colemannatural.com), hormone free meat, if you are going to eat it.

Havit Raw Foods (www.bluemountainorganics.com), 540-745-5040.

Organic Direct (www.organicdirect.com).

Vital Choice—Wild Alaskan seafood. 866-482-5887

Cancer Conquest video- order it on www.burtongoldberg.com. $19.99 for 1 week online access and $39,99 for 1 week online access and DVD by mail.

HealthMaster blender by Montel Williams (www.myhealthmaster.com).

The Pampered Patient (www.thepamperedpatient.com), order gift baskets for cancer patients.

Cottage Dreams (www.cottagedreams.ca), residents in Ontario Canada with cancer can apply for a free vacation at a cottage with family.

Cancer Survivor Beauty and Support Day (www.cancersurvivorbeautyandsupportday.org), the first Tuesday in June cancer survivors get free spa services!

Acknowledgments

I thank my mother Miriam, for bringing me into this world, talking to me on a daily basis throughout treatment, visiting every Friday, and helping us support our kids throughout this journey. Her strength with her own Parkinson's was inspiring.

I thank my father Marc and his wife, Lana, for visiting every Sunday, gifting me with boxes of special water for cancer, UV clothing so I could walk the beach, car service vouchers, financial support, and love and encouragement.

I thank my mother-in-law Katherine Sherman for babysitting her grandchildren many weekends without which the writing of this book would not have been possible. Writing it helped me make sense of my own journey and hopefully it will help other women facing breast cancer and illness be successful on this path. We all thank you with love!

I thank my husband, Ian, for attending most of my chemotherapy treatments with me, being the person I came home to on a daily basis, being my friend, lover, and soul mate, and for loving me even when I was bald and tired.

I thank my children Sera and Noble for their unconditional joy and love. I want to have a long life with you guys!

I thank Christopher Dilts for being my Spiritual mentor when I needed support and for teaching me the next level of healing for myself and others. Thank you so much for being my earth angel Christopher! Words can never convey what this means to me.

I thank my sister Avra and her boyfriend Albert for visiting me twice when I was diagnosed and sending me love and encouragement.

I thank Dan Koiffman of Workaholics Anonymous, my neighbor and diet coach for putting up with me and for all the great tips!

I thank Kenzi for her beautiful henna crown!

I thank our nanny Rhonda and our babysitter Kim for providing continuity and care for our children when I was at the hospital or at work.

I thank Dr. Sacchini at Sloan Kettering hospital for performing the lumpectomy, Dr. Malamud for helping me through chemotherapy, and Dr. Paula Klein for subbing the day I had to stay late for chemotherapy.

I thank Dr. Rescignio, my radiologist, for his support, his many conversations about my book, his flexibility in helping me get through 33 daily radiation treatments and his wonderful staff.

I thank Dr. Salerno at the Salerno Center for helping me to build my immune system and overall health after treatment.

I thank Susan Silberstein at BeatCancer.org for her great advice.

I thank my friends Aida, Jill, Karen, Ana, Leigh and Rachel and my new cancer friend Jen.

I thank my mentors and consultants including Dr. Terri Kennedy, Dr. Vargas and Dr. Bruce Lackie.

I thank Gilda, my mom's assistant and our family friend, for her encouragement and humor.

I thank Sarah at Neshama Preschool for loving, inspiring, and educating our son.

I thank my editor Margie Holt Smith, a volunteer editor from Visible Ink and Judith Kelman for founding it. Thanks also to Wendy Thorton whom I hired as an editor through elance and Julie Clayton for her editing flair.

I thank Emily Rubin for her free writers series for cancer survivors at Beth Israel.

I thank my book designer Sara Blum who is wonderful to partner with and a real talent!

Thanks to my neighbors and people in my building. Sherry, Ruth, Barbara, Risa and Svetlana for asking how I am and the maintenance men like Pete, Raymond and Neville for saying I look great bald and checking on me. It makes a difference.

I thank the whole gang at MNA, including Bill, Leah, Jessica, Beeba, Stephanie, Tom and everyone for their love and Seabreeze car service for getting me to the hospital and work in time every morning.

I thank my book reviewers who took time out of their busy schedule to read my work and offer an endorsement . It made me feel part of a community of healers who really care.

I thank my coaching and psychotherapy clients for helping me learn as a healer.

I thank Stage 2 breast cancer for making me think about what I still wanted to do in my life and being my guide.

I thank the Divine and my angels for giving me unconditional love when I needed it most and the beach near for helping to heal me. Lastly, I thank Ana Negron for her inspiring Forword, her vitality, radiance, friendship and participation in this project.

I thank Ray Foley for his beautiful pictures.

I thank my Indiegogo helpers including Zoe Schneider, Nellie Escalante, Maria Voulamandis, Nellie Dumburger, Rachel Vine, Dave Powell, Skye Gabel, Miriam Kove, Marc Kouffman, Samantha Jones, Francine Berkowitz, Aida Reyes, Leigh Woods, Ruth Torres and Ian Sherman and all the people who spread the word to make this dream a reality and help women going through this. God bless you for your generous hearts.

APPENDIX A

Reaching Out to Organizations for Financial Help

Patient Advocate Foundation (www.patientadvocate.org) Assists people with medical debt crisis, insurance access issues, job retention issues. 800-532-5274.

Co-Pay Relief Program (www.copays.org) Provides financial support to insured patients. There is a web application or call 866-512-3861.

Healthwell Foundation (www.healthwellfoundation.org) They address patients with insurance who can't afford co-pays or premiums for their medical insurance. 800-675-8416.

Modest Needs (www.modestneeds.org) The maximum grant they provide is either $1000 or 7.5% of your household's verifiable income, whichever is greater. 212-463-7042.

Patient Access Network Foundation (www.panfoundation.org) They facilitate treatment for patients with life threatening illnesses. You must be insured to use their services. Patient's income must be a designated percentage of the Federal Poverty level. For online application: www.panfoundation.org/fundingapplication/patientEnrollment.php. 866-316-7263.

Team Continuum (www.teamcontinuum.net) They help with things that ease the burdens of everyday treatment assisting with bills, rent, tutoring, small toys, transportation and other incidental needs that arise. To apply online: www.teamcontinuum.net/apply_for_a_grant or call 212-951-7201. For application assistance by phone call 917-595-4196.

Cancer Fund of America, Inc. (www.cfoa.org) They send personal care products like vitamins, gift boxes, fans, lotions, ointments, food and non prescription medicine. 800-578-5284.

National Foundation for Credit Counseling (www.debtadvice.org) They advise you on your money and debt. To find a counselor call 800-388-2227.

Community Service Society of New York (www.cssny.org) They help people get jobs through technical assistance. 212-614-5586.

Lifewise Family Financial Security provide credit for individuals and families facing life-threatening illnesses. They have a resource guide with resources too and a staff of oncology nurses to answer medical, financial and insurance questions. 800-219-7385.

Livestrong can help you if you are underinsured or uninsured. 855-220-7777.

This is a good start. I did not need to use this list yet as I was ultimately able to work something out with Sloan Kettering. But, should your hospital not work with you, or should you still need help with co-pays despite your insurance, here are some options. I don't know how hefty the time and paperwork is but it's always helpful to have support and free stuff so you decide if it is worth it and you have the energy to pursue it.

APPENDIX B

The Cancer Organizations & Magazines

Beat Cancer (www.beatcancer.org), Director: Susan Silberstein

You Can Thrive (www.youcanthrive.org), Director: Luana DeAngelis

Cancer Care (www.cancercare.org)

Henna Heals (www.hennaheals.ca)

Look Good, Feel Better (lookgoodfeelbetter.org) This is a two-hour class that teaches you to do your eyebrows and apply makeup for your coloring. They have it at most hospitals. Call them at 1-800-395-LOOK

Visible Ink (www.visibleinkmskcc.org) Writing program at Sloan Kettering. Contact Judith Kelman at judith.kelman@gmail.com

Gilda's Club (www.gildasclubnyc.org)

Love Your Transformation (www.lytnyc.com) for colonics in Manhattan

National Breast Cancer Foundation, Inc.
(www.nationalbreastcancer.org)

National Cancer Institute (www.cancer.gov)

American Cancer Society (www.cancer.org)

Breast Cancer Fund (www.breastcancerfund.org)

Breast Cancer Options (www.breastcanceroptions.org) They put out a great annual calendar and offer a free sleep away camp for kids of parents with breast cancer, called *Camp Lightheart.* See their website for more information.

Share (www.sharecancersupport.org)

National Coalition for Cancer Survivorship
(www.canceradvocacy.org)

Susan Komen Breast Cancer Foundation (ww5.komen.org)
1-800-IM AWARE.

Karen Wellington Foundation for LIVING with Breast Cancer
(www.karenwellingtonfoundation.org) an organization in honor of Karen Wellington that gives vacations to cancer survivors.

Send Me On Vacation (www.sendmeonvacation.org) an organization that picks some cancer survivors and awards them up to $1500 for a vacation.

Stowe Weekend of Hope (www.stowehope.org) a weekend of free hotels and workshops in Vermont for cancer survivors. This year it's in May 2013 and you can register in February.

Cancer Hope Network (www.cancerhopenetwork.org)
877-HOPENET

Cancer Legal Resource Center (www.disabilityrightslegalcenter.org/cancer-legal-resource-center)

Know Cancer (www.knowcancer.com)

Locks of Love (www.locksoflove.org)

Bikur Cholim Partners in Health (www.bikurcholim.com) is an organization that arranges for people to travel to hospitals, nursing homes or other places to visit ill, home-bound or distressed people. These typically are Jewish organizations that believe that Bikur Cholim is both a religious and societal obligation. Some organizations have branched out to include other medical services. They organize volunteers to visit sick, elderly, recovering or home-bound people in many different venues, such as hospitals, nursing homes, rehabilitation centers and private homes. In addition to visits, volunteers will sometimes take the person on errands or to some other activity. Sometimes these visits and trips are supplemented by phone calls and other ways of keeping in touch with the sick or recovering person. These visits and other activities are meant to lift their spirits and reassure them that people care about them. Contact: 25 Robert Pitt Drive Suite 101, Monsey, NY 10952, phone: 845.425.7877, fax: 845.425.5061, email: bcinfo@bikurcholim.org, emergency hotline: 845.425.4567

Cancer and Careers (www.cancerandcareers.org) living and working with cancer

Chemo Angels (www.chemoangels.net) they send things to encourage you

Young Survival Coalition (www.youngsurvival.org) help for younger patients

Layers Of Love (www.layersoflove.net) supplies free fleece blankets to chemo patients. On Facebook: https://www.facebook.com/LayersofLoveComfortingChemotherapyPatients

Spirit Jump (www.spiritjump.org) is a grassroots non-profit organization with a mission to provide hope and comfort to the many men, women and children battling cancer. Spirit Jump accomplishes this by providing uplifting cards and inspirational gifts during this most difficult time. Email: needaspiritjump@spiritjump.com

FertileHope (www.fertilehope.com) is dedicated to providing reproductive information, support and hope to cancer patients and survivors whose medical treatments present the risk of infertility. If you have fertility-related questions or would like more information related to the Sharing Hope financial assistance program, you can complete an online intake form for the LIVESTRONG Navigation Services program at www.livestrong.org/Get-Help/Get-One-On-One-Support or if you'd like to speak with someone directly, call 855.220.7777.

Cookies for Kids' Cancer (www.cookiesforkidscancer.org) an organization that raises money for kids with cancer.

Miracle House (www.miraclehouse.org) provides a place for patients and caregivers to stay in Manhattan for $50 a night with a private bedroom and a shared living room.

Life Extension Foundation (www.lef.org/goodhealth) They test your hormone levels. 888-884-3666.

Chemosensitivity Testing

Biofocus Institute for Laboratory Medicine, email: prix@biofocus.de
Research Genetic Cancer Center, email: jpapasot@doctors.org.uk

Testing for Nutritional Deficiencies

Genovia Diagnostics (www.gdx.net), 800-522-4762

CANCER MAGAZINES & EZINES

Cure Magazine

Cancer Today Magazine

Living with Cancer

Breast Cancer Wellness

Women & Cancer Magazine

Women

4Wholeness.com

Healtoday.com

ican4u.com

Cancerwise.org

Coping With Cancer 615-791-3859

cfthrive.com

breastcancerwellness.org

Insight

waitingroommagazine.com

MAMM (www.mamm.com)

APPENDIX C

The Healers & Helpers in this Book

Christopher Dilts spiritual counselor
www.askanangel.org

Dr. Terri Kennedy life coach
www.drterrikennedy.com

Dan Koiffman health coach
www.workaholicworkouts.com

You Can Thrive
nonprofit for alternative healing for breast cancer patients
www.youcanthrive.com

LaUna Huffines
Angel tapes for healing, sleep and relaxation
www.healingwithlight.org

Bradley Hess energy healer with a center called 'Intuitive Energy' in Media, PA.
www.intuitiveenergy.com

Tom Cratsley cellular reconstruction
tom@tomcratsley.com, 716-595-3551

Michelle WhiteDove psychic
www.michellewhitedove.com, 952-981-2828

Dr. Ana Negron doctor and nutritional consultant
www.greensonabudget.com

Dr. Nicholas Gonzalez a program with diet, supplementation & detoxification in NYC
www.dr-gonzalez.com, 212-213-3337

Gerson Institute
www.gerson.org, 619-685-5353

Kenzi henna designer
(can do henna crowns)
www.kenzi.com

Tari Prinster yoga teacher who focuses on cancer survivors
y4c.com or www.tariprinster.com

Eloise De Leon
www.insightandjoy.com, eloise@insightandjoy.com

Katie Lamb
www.touchofhopefromthehealing.com,
katie@touchofhope@yahoo.com, 208-529-6633

Den Pikey virtual assistant
www.denpikey.com

Ray Foley photographer
(he can take photos of your cancer experience)
www.grain-pictures.com

Nick and Jessica Ortner are great teachers in Tapping
www.thetappingsolution.com.

Joyce Hawkes
www.celllevelhealing.com

The Salerno Center
www.salernocenter.com

APPENDIX D

A Blood Count Guide & Glossary for Chemotherapy

ALT: alanine trasmamisase is an ensyme in the liver, heart, muscles and kidneys. This is sometimes used to diagnose kidney disease.

AST: aspartate transmainase helps the body metabolize glucose and when cells are injured or die AST is released into the blood stream. It measures the presence of damaged cells so it's a clue about how treatment is going.

LD: lactic acid dehydrenase is an enzyme in cell, especially in the kidney, liver, brain, lungs, heart and skeletal muscles. It's useful to monitor organs.

LIPPOPROTEIN TESTS

Cholesterol: related to heart disease and atheroskeletososis.

Triglycerides: test to see how the body metabolizes fats. It's better to do when fasting.

Lipoprotein Electrophoresis: measures various lipoproteins in the blood.

TUMOR MARKERS

CEA: this is found in 60% of all breast cancer tumors in humans. It is a measure used to monitor chemotherapy.

HER2: this is a genetic mutation that can be over expressed and isn't common. 30% of breast cancer patients are HER2 positive.

About the Author

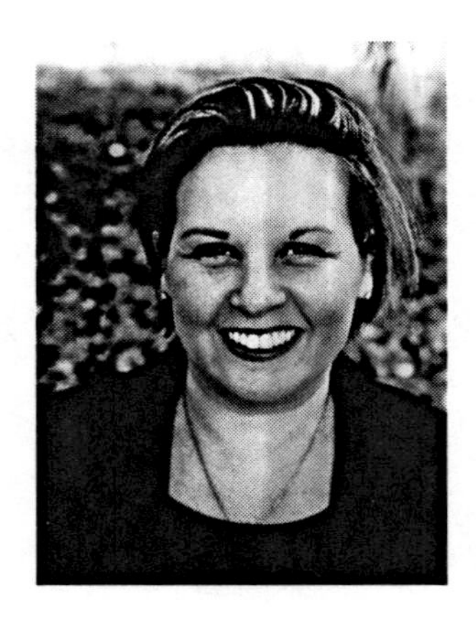

Paulette Kouffman Sherman is a breast cancer survivor, wife, mother of two, psychologist, coach, author, speaker and teacher. She loves the beach, singing, writing, spirituality and learning.

Professionally she is a Licensed Psychologist with concentrations in school psychology and family therapy, a certified empowerment coach, an author, teacher and speaker. She has worked as a healer in a variety of settings including high schools, universities, hospitals, partial programs, nursing homes, group and private psychotherapy practices and nursery lab schools. Practices have included the Brooklyn Center for Families in Crisis, Psychological Services & Human Development Center, LaSalle University Counseling Center, Elwyn, Inc., Silberman Center, Crozer-Chester Hospital, Delaware County Intermediate Unit, Widener Lab School, Christiana Hospital, Media Child Guidance, Arlington Children's Center, Bellevue Hospital Therapeutic Nursery, and Hassenfeld Children's Center for Oncology & Blood Diseases. She has worked with patients with a range of issues, including depression, anxiety, career issues, familial and personal struggles and losses.

Dr. Sherman has specialized in relationship issues and is the author of *Dating From the Inside Out* published by Atria Books. She's also the Director of *My Dating School* in New York City and has been a frequent speaker at *The Learning Annex*. Dr. Sherman writes a column as the NY Love Examiner, and has been an expert on the *CBS Early Show*, the *AM Northwest Early Show* and the *Curtis Sliwa* show on 77WABC. She has been quoted as a relationship expert or interviewed in over 30 outlets such as *MSN.com*, *USA Weekend*, the *NY Post*, *Crains*, *Newsweek*, *Lifetime.com*, *More*, *Match.com*, *Foxnews.com*, *FoxBusiness*, *Better Homes & Gardens*, *Reader's Digest*, *Redbook*, *Glamour*, *Forbes*, *Woman's Day*, *Metro newspapers*, *Men's Health*, *True Story*, *Seventeen*, *Complete Woman* magazines, *The Huffington Post* and *The New York Times*. She lives in Brooklyn with her husband and two children.

IF YOU LIKE WHAT YOU JUST READ AND WANT TO LEARN MORE . . .

Other Books by Dr. Paulette Kouffman Sherman

4 Volume Set: "Your Cancer Path"

My Quick Guide Through Breast Cancer: Diagnosis, Surgery, Chemo & Radiation (Volume 1)

The Cancer Path: A Spiritual Journey Into Healing Wholeness & Love (Volume 2)

My Date With Cancer: 21 Spiritual Lessons (Volume 3)

The Create Your Own Cancer Path Workbook (Volume 4)

Dating & Relationship Books

When Mars Women Date: How Career Women Can Love Themselves Into the Relationship of Their Dreams

Dating from the Inside Out: How to Use the Law of Attraction in Matters of the Heart

A Shared Vision: 100 Conversations to Co-Create the Relationship of Your Dreams

100 Ways to Treat Your Mate like Royalty: Under $10

Children's Books

Shekhina

You can order these books through my website www.parachutejump-publishing or on Amazon. Look for 15 more books to come in this Legacy project. You can go to my website to make a donation to my Legacy Project or email me about it at kpaulet@verizon.net.

Dr. Kouffman Sherman will also be offering groups, teleclasses and psychotherapy for cancer patients as a psychologist. Contact her to learn more at www.thecancerpath.com! You can see video clips about The Cancer Path topics at www.youtube.com/user/TheCancerPath!

You can also visit Dr. Paulette Kouffman Sherman's other website, My Dating School, for information on dating coaching. There may be an upcoming book on dating with cancer as well! You can email Paulette at kpaulet@verizon.net. See you soon!

Dr. Sherman's Other Websites:

www.thecancerpath.com
www.parachutejumppublishing.com
www.mydatingschool.com
www.whenmarswomendate.com
www.PauletteSherman.com

CPSIA information can be obtained
at www.ICGtesting.com
Printed in the USA
EDOW031328020513
1421ED

9 780985 246945